The lovecare Effect

How Planning in Advance Can Save Your Life

Lee Lambert

The Lovecare Effect: How Planning in Advance Can Save Your Life

By Lee Lambert

Copyright © 2023 Lee Lambert

All rights reserved. No part of this book may be reproduced or transmitted in any form or by any means, either in print or electronically without written permission from the author, except for brief quotations in book reviews or news articles.

Published by Legacy Press Books
A subsidiary of S & P Productions, Inc.
311 Main Street, Suite D
El Segundo, CA 90245
310-640-8885
www.legacypressbooks.com

Published and Printed in the United States of America

ISBN: 978-1-7329566-4-3

The content contained in The Lovecare Effect: How Planning in Advance Can Save Your Life, is for informational purposes only. The content is not intended to be a substitute for medical, professional, or psychological advice, diagnosis, or treatment. Always seek the advice of your physician or other qualified healthcare providers and professionals with any questions you may have regarding medical, mental health, legal or financial concerns. Always seek the advice of qualified professionals in matters relating to any finance or business undertakings.

Dedication

I dedicate this book to my father. Without sharing this precious time together at the end, my life would have never evolved as it did. He saved me. At the end of the day, he is a testament to the truth of how powerful love is. When nothing is left; not money, not things, when all control is lost and everything is gone, love shines like a brilliant star guiding you back home.

I also want to dedicate it to caregivers everywhere whether they be future, current or caregivers whose loved ones have already passed on. None of us will ever be the same person as the one who said yes when it was our turn. There is no more enriching or revealing experience than the loss of a parent over time. Whatever we are, it all started with them.

It's a time to weep and yet a time of pure joy where love trumps all.

Daddy

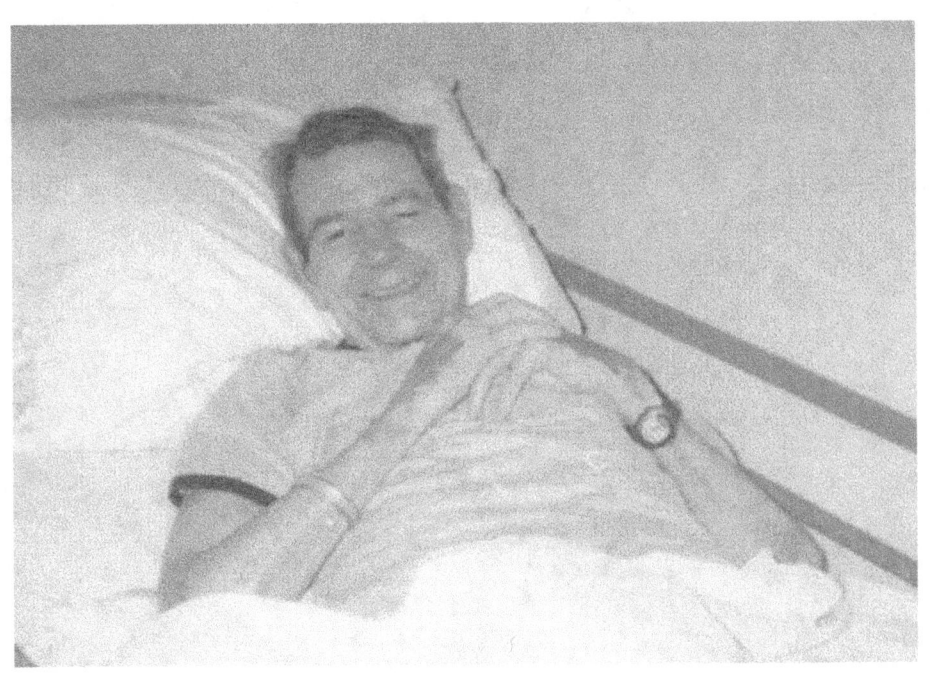

1923 – 2007

Alzheimer's Disease

Table of Contents

Introduction i

About the Author v

Chapter 1 Don't Wait for an Emergency to Plan 1

Chapter 2 Get a Medical Evaluation - Hope Is Not a Strategy 10

Chapter 3 Have the Conversation 14

Chapter 4 Put Safety Practices in Place 21

Chapter 5 Create a Comprehensive Plan 28

Chapter 6 How Does Cognitive Dissonance Threaten Your Success 35

Chapter 7 The Checklist 41

Chapter 8 Questions to Ask Yourself Before Becoming The Primary Caregiver 48

Chapter 9 A Change in Perspective 54

Chapter 10 Start Monitoring Your Loved One Early .. 60

Chapter 11 Understanding the Big Picture 69

Chapter 12 Be "Option Ready" 73

Chapter 13 Organize Your Team 78

Chapter 14 Building Resilience for the Caregiving Marathon 82

Chapter 15 Plan the Funeral While Still Healthy 90

Chapter 16 Take Time to Heal 94

Introduction

Caregiving is a unique time in life when the past, present and who you will become after, converge. It's not a sprint, it's a marathon in many ways.

It can devastate you or teach you to trust life. It's a time for reevaluating what's important. It's a time of letting go. It's a painful gift that can transform grief into new meaning and purpose if you allow it.

Caregiving is not something you do, it's something you live. You may not know this until you step through that door. That's why it's important to plan in advance because this will be one of the most important jobs you will ever do.
If you're caregiving now, what will you learn and more importantly, what will you do with it?

I was my father's caregiver for 15 years. He had Alzheimer's disease. It was the hardest and the sweetest time of my life.

That's why I created an end-to-end system for the comprehensive planning that's needed for all stages of care, so that you will not have to make the same mistakes I made.

This book is not only about the logistics of what makes caregiving successful, it's also about how loss can teach us how precious life is.

Just like the flapping wings of a butterfly can be felt around the world, the small changes we make while caregiving can transform the whole experience.

Love is in the details ...

lovecare

About the Author

You may think that I was sitting around trying to figure out what to do with my life when I took on the responsibility of caring for my father. It was a huge decision under the best circumstances. But actually, it turned out not to be not such a huge decision after all. It didn't matter what effect it might have on my life. What mattered was that he needed me.

I dropped everything and headed for Alabama with two trucks and a few big guys. Within one day, we had loaded up his whole life and off we went, back from whence we came, Atlanta.

I had moved there after college to pursue a career in design after launching a tennis shop at a local club and getting great design reviews. Although I probably should have pursued a business degree instead, I'm sure that path would not have led me to where I am now.

I was running a manufacturing company with over 80 people who depended on me. Like many entrepreneurs, the staff was lean and as an owner, you had to be everywhere, think on your feet and hope that God was watching over you.

Although successful, it was necessary to maintain tight controls on everything. This takes a human toll over time. To be honest, I was already burned out before my father even arrived. In fact, if it were not for him, I might not have even survived the stressful life I was living.

I thought the broad range of experience over the evolution of my career in design, construction, furniture and real estate would come in handy as I transitioned out of my company to care for my father. However, as grief took over, I was never able to transition as easily as I thought into a less demanding, smaller business. Over time, I found it harder and harder to cope, feeling more overwhelmed each day until in the end, I lost everything. But I have to say, that this seemingly horrible outcome was a blessing in disguise.

It was only afterward, when I began to write about what had happened, that I was able to transform my grief into new meaning and purpose. It became my single focus to make sure that no one else would have to go through what I went through. I began to develop an entire system for other caregivers to know what to do and when to do it. Unlike me, they would have a chance to live their own lives more normally during the care of a loved one, creating a legacy to be proud of instead of spiraling down like I did.

However, the process of caring for my father taught me everything about what I had been missing in my life and why I had failed at the one thing everyone has to face at some point, knowing who they really are.

Loss puts everything into perspective. It clarifies what's most important. It simplifies life and it forces you to stand in the void of the unknown every day and trust something bigger than yourself.

And the pain makes you stronger.

What if …

… your father fell?

… and could no longer live alone?

…where would he go?

…how would you take care of him?

With one fall, you could become a caregiver overnight!

That's what happened to me and my father. He became ill with Alzheimer's and I became his caregiver for the next 15 years.

Over 10,000 people are turning 65 every day and there are no longer enough nurses or facilities to handle their care.

Don't make the same mistakes I did. **Plan now,** before crisis happens.

I'm here to show you how.

See my video story at caregivingoutloud.com

Chapter 1
Don't Wait for an Emergency to Plan

"Life's challenges are not supposed to paralyze you; they're supposed to help you discover who you are."
- Bernice Johnson Reagon

Are You Ready for the Surprise Phone Call?

Imagine.....getting that call. A neighbor has just found your father on the kitchen floor, unable to get up. He's been lying there since early morning when he went to make breakfast. It's now 4:00 in the afternoon.

Heartbroken, you think of him lying there all alone for so long with no way to call for help. You jump in the car and rush to meet the ambulance at the hospital, not knowing what you might find. Difficult to think straight, you may even feel a little guilty that you didn't do more to somehow to prevent this from happening. Totally unprepared for what's about to unfold, you still wonder why you didn't see it coming.

After reviewing your father's condition, the doctor tells you, "He's very confused, weak, and dehydrated, but he'll be okay. However, he cannot go back home to live alone."

You've had nightmares about this moment, hearing those words, and yet you've done nothing to prepare for it. Your father is not dying; he's aging.

You have just become a caregiver overnight!

An emergency is often the most common doorway through which most of us enter the caregiving journey. If you waited for an emergency to happen and found yourself overwhelmed by the prospect—not knowing what to do next—you are not alone!

But you can change everything from this point forward by planning in advance.

Where would your father go if he could no longer live alone?

Although the specifics of each situation are different (from a fall to a heart attack), most of us wait for an emergency to act. This unexpected event is a wake-up call to the beginning stages of a loved one's decline. However, no matter what the circumstances, we all tend to react in surprise, as if this day was never going to actually come.

It boils down to the important question of where your parents will go to live, not *if* but *when* they can no longer live by themselves. In an emergency, you may have only two to three days to plan before they're released from the hospital. However, this is not the only question that needs to be answered. Caregiving is a commitment that can rock your world if you have not created a comprehensive plan. Take it from me.

Unfortunately, many of us find ourselves planning for long-term care in the emergency room, making snap decisions that may not work.

So, let's get started ...

Do You Know the Answers to These Five Questions?

- Do you know where your parent's financial information is?
- Do you know what their wishes are?
- Do you have legal authority to act on their behalf?
- Do you know how you will pay for their care?
- What kind of insurance policies do they have?

Why Do We Wait for an Emergency to Plan?

A Harvard study found that the number one reason why people don't plan in advance is **denial.**

Denial is the first stage of grief when someone dies. But when a loved one doesn't die but rather declines over time, denial can permeate every stage of their care, impeding you from giving them the assistance they need and deserve along the way. It's a coping mechanism we use to deal with a loss we cannot emotionally accept. We all do it!

Denial can become an existential threat to a loved one's safety and quality of life if not dealt with effectively. It creates inaction and can stop families from preventing unnecessary crises from happening over and over. It can also keep your life in turmoil, not knowing what to expect and never being prepared for what happens during the process of decline.

A fact-based approach is essential and requires consistent objectivity. But how do you maintain objectivity throughout such a challenging and highly emotional time? The intricacies of this question are what this book is all about. In fact, it's for this specific reason that I created a system of checks and balances that you can put in place ahead of time for navigating the important decisions and to help deal with the emotional impact that can potentially interfere with the process.

Don't Let Caregiving Become the "Long Emergency"

I call caregiving the long emergency because many of us go from one emergency to another throughout every stage of care without a plan. Instead, we play Whack-a-Mole with our loved one's care, catching our breath in between crises and hoping somehow to magically elude future events.

That's why caregivers not only need a reality check, but a system of reality checks to keep themselves from lapsing into denial. In fact, the lovecare system is specifically designed to keep you from doing the same thing over and over, expecting different results. Sound familiar?

The initial emergency often sets up a chain reaction of crisis management that continues if you don't come to terms with what this challenge means for your life, and what it will require. Whether you are remote, estranged, have a busy life, or even have a good relationship, caregiving a loved one is a crossroads where you must prioritize what's important.

How Can an Emergency Help You to Mitigate Future Risks?

Never let a crisis go to waste! An emergency is a crisis, yes. But if you pay attention there's a lot you can learn from it. It's a time when the experts are laser focused on your loved ones most pressing needs. Their condition is being reevaluated, and their treatment adjusted. New medical information will help you decide whether to care for them at home, what you need to monitor or if a move to a facility may be in their best interest. It's a time to reset the parameters so that your loved one's highest quality of life is protected for as long as possible. Often, an emergency can cast a fresh perspective on what is needed to make them more comfortable and to keep them safe from future events.

However, if you're paralyzed by emotion, you may miss the opportunity for important insights to be gained or forget to share what you have observed with the doctor. You are your loved one's voice now. Your role is to make sure that your loved one is getting the best possible care and achieving the best possible outcomes. Anything short of being fully present for this responsibility will not get the outcomes your loved one deserves.

I'm Here to Help You Do That Job!

Quality of life is fragile. One event can easily develop into a snowball from which your loved one may never recover. That's why staying ahead of their decline and being proactive is so important.

My Aunt's Story

Just before Thanksgiving, my aunt, a vibrant 84-year-old, turned slightly the wrong way while getting into bed at the Independent Living Facility where she was living. She fell, breaking her hip. It was tragic, but unfortunately not uncommon.

Her attitude was incredible as she fought through physical therapy for almost three months. But the person I was more worried about was my uncle, who after more than 60 years of marriage, never left her side. This included sleeping upright in a chair, by her side, most of the time.

Their two adult children, now fifty-something with grown kids of their own, were also there. Both were familiar with the statistics on the unlikely recovery from a broken hip at her age. Encouragement was the most important medicine at this point. However, my aunt was the one doing the encouraging, cracking jokes and assuring us that she wasn't going anywhere.

We were beginning to feel just as confident as she was, as her release date was approaching, until we got some additional news. Her immune system had become so compromised during this setback that her cancer from 30 years prior, had now returned.

When my aunt got this news, she decided that it was her time to go. I remember when my father decided it was his time. He died three days later, the exact amount of time it took my aunt. Neither she nor my father knew the meaning of giving up. Both had led rich lives, full of challenges and accomplishments. They were courageous by any standard. However, they both knew when it was their time.

Falls are the number one injury leading to premature death of the elderly. You can see how things can snowball, going from an active functioning life to finding oneself bedridden and compromised. It's critical to do everything possible to prevent falls from happening during every stage of care.

Hip Fracture Prevention Checklist

- ☐ Exercise regularly
- ☐ Include weight-bearing exercises
- ☐ Increase leg strength and improve balance
- ☐ Identify medicines with side effects of dizziness or drowsiness
- ☐ Make home safety improvements
- ☐ Adequate intake of calcium and vitamin D

- ☐ Get screened and treated for osteoporosis
- ☐ Keep your home well-lit
- ☐ Shoes should have nonskid soles
- ☐ Remove electrical cords from walking areas
- ☐ Remove stools and step ladders
- ☐ Avoid waxing the floors
- ☐ Sidewalks, walkways, stairs should be in good repair with even (flat), nonslip surfaces
- ☐ Sore feet, foot pain and corns may provoke falls

Checklist of Common Causes of Nursing Home Falls

- ☐ Muscle weakness and walking or gait problems cause 24% of falls.
- ☐ Environmental hazards in nursing homes cause 16-27% of falls due to wet floors, poor lighting, incorrect bed height, improperly fitted or maintained wheelchairs, to name a few.
- ☐ Fall risk is significantly elevated during the three days following any change in medications such as sedatives and anti-anxiety drugs.
- ☐ Poor foot care, poorly fitting shoes, improper or incorrect use of walking aids all contribute to nursing home falls.

Preventing Falls in Nursing Homes Checklist

- ☐ Identify and assess risk factors
- ☐ Make changes to the environment
- ☐ Provide hip pads
- ☐ Exercise programs
- ☐ Vitamin D
- ☐ Teach residents to avoid potentially hazardous situations

Use the Emergency to Begin Developing Your Comprehensive Plan

The family caregiver is the tip of the spear. You will need every tool in the toolbox to be successful. Successful caregiving comes down to two important things:

- Monitoring your loved one for changes in condition
- Objective fact-based decision-making

Effective methods for handling both are essential to create successful outcomes and to prevent ongoing crises. If you are not on top of your loved one's condition, you cannot take the necessary action to maintain their quality of life. If your emotions interfere with your objectivity, poor decisions can lead to do-overs—wasting precious resources and endangering your loved one's comfort, safety, and ultimately, their life. Both factors impact your ability to be successful in achieving good outcomes.

I designed each tool in the system with the assumption that you are probably busy, distracted from time to time, most likely emotional, and at times overwhelmed. After all, you have your own life to live with an entirely separate set of challenges to face every day. And yet, you want to do your best job, not just some of the time, but all the time. It matters! Considering the array of emotions you may feel from one day to the next, I think it's impossible to expect yourself to maintain the necessary objectivity required for making good decisions on a consistent basis. Let's face it, we're all human.

Having a guide to see the big picture so that you can understand what to do and when to do it is incredibly helpful when you're handling a major issue like long-term care for the first time. No matter how smart you are, you don't know what you don't know.

Besides, with everything else going on, it's nice to be able to just **follow instructions**.

Go to **caregivingoutloud.com** to take the **Emergency Course NOW!**

Pause and Reflect

- Where would your parent go if they could no longer live alone?

- Are you waiting for an emergency to plan?

- Without planning, an emergency can put in motion a perpetual mode of crisis management.

- You can learn a lot from the emergency if you pay attention and know what to ask.

Are you ready for the surprise phone call?

Chapter 2
Get a Medical Evaluation -
Hope Is Not a Strategy

"We live in a fantasy world, a world of illusion. The great task in life is to find reality."

– Iris Murdoch

What is Your Loved One's Current Medical Condition?

The medical evaluation will give you a baseline from which to measure all future changes in condition. Clarity, not hope, is the basis for taking effective action. You can hope that they will be okay or fear that they will not, but both can keep you from giving them the clear-thinking support that they require. Pursuing the facts objectively is the only path toward meeting their needs.

A clear understanding of your loved one's current condition reveals several important things.

- Current needs
- Expectations for the future
- Type of planning required

Acting on this information as early as possible will yield the best results. The medical evaluation can take the form of a standard annual check-up. Your loved one may seem fine, but even if they seem okay, being proactive may uncover an underlying condition that hasn't yet presented itself. If so, you may have just avoided a trip to the emergency room without even knowing it.

Or perhaps you observe some initial signs of decline where you feel a higher sense of urgency to evaluate what may be developing. By the time you notice something, often the issue is more advanced than you realized. In any case, the medical evaluation is a proactive measure that can get the facts clearly on the table, allowing you and your family to understand the parameters of your loved one's current health. It also provides you with a window of time to begin planning for the future.

What Are Your Loved One's Current Needs?

Your loved one's independence is crucial, but their safety is just as important. Try putting yourself in their shoes before suggesting solutions. Imagine if it were your own life and independence being decided upon and see if the solution you have presented has considered both safety and respected their need for freedom.

The medical evaluation may show that they're doing great. Whew, what a relief, right? Not so fast! This is their current status, meaning *at the moment*. They're aging and will need to be monitored carefully even if there are no immediate issues to be addressed. In fact, this can be one of the most important times. Be careful not to celebrate the good news, put it in a drawer, and take your eye off the ball. Proper monitoring is critical for preventing unnecessary crises going forward. If there are any current concerns that need attention, your doctor should explain exactly how to address them.

- Does your loved one need a new medication?
- How closely do they need to be monitored?
- Would medical equipment be helpful?
- Do they need professional help at home?
- Is it time to ask the "Big Questions"?

Should they be driving?

Should they be cooking?

Should they be living alone?

What Can You Expect in the Future?

Ask how serious the concern is and how the doctor expects it to progress over time. This information will help you with two important things.

- Your planning window
- What to monitor

Remember that your life will be impacted more and more as your loved one declines. Knowing where things stand at all times is the best form of mitigation that you can use to keep living your life as normally as possible.

Decline Drives Financial Planning

How you plan may or may not depend on a specific condition. Whether the decline is due to aging or a chronic disease, they both share a similar planning process, even if the specific condition may be different. All stages of decline contain some unknowns. However, your loved one's ongoing need for increased care will require the family to plan how to pay for each stage. Homecare can help you to stretch resources; the longer you can care for them at home the more you can save for future care. Their decline and need for increased care will create the projects, moves, and purchases that will drive your financial planning.

Set Up Your Medical Manager

The medical evaluation is the perfect time to set up your Medical Manager. Everything will need to be documented in order to measure all future changes in condition. This is key for responding to their ongoing needs with incremental adjustments or a move for increased care. Maintaining their safety and quality of life will extend your ability to keep them at home for as long as possible.

Learn how to set up your Medical Manager in the Medical Module.

**GET YOUR SIGNS OF DECLINE CHECKLIST
@caregivingoutloud.com**

Pause and Reflect

- Have you noticed any signs of decline?

- Have you asked the "Big Questions"?

- Do you know what your loved one's current needs are?

- Are you putting off taking your loved one for a medical evaluation?

Be proactive and learn how to set up your Medical Manager now!

Chapter 3
Have the Conversation

"A dysfunctional family is any family with more than one person in it."

- Mary Karr

Going Back Home: How Do You Make Good Decisions as a Family?

Having a structured process to follow for family conversations is key to making good decisions regarding the care and assistance of your loved one as they age. Decisions must be measurable while taking into consideration the impact they will have on the overall plan. They cannot be made emotionally or deterred by family dynamics or unclear objectives.

Although each family is different, most have a complicated history that tends to unravel during the challenges of long-term care. Most of us experience this on a very personal level. The process of making decisions together as adults can feel like you're in effect, "going back home." Unresolved issues from years past may reappear as if it were yesterday. However, despite the possibly uncomfortable process, you may be surprised to find that it can also be one of the most insightful times of your life. In fact, these caregiving challenges can help you to grow personally and the family to grow closer.

So, let's get started!

How Do You Stay Objective as a Family?

One of the key tests each family faces to one degree or another is how to stay objective. There are many challenges that can make this difficult.

Logistical Challenges

There are personal distractions that keep you from being fully present.

- Career
- Kids
- Time Restraints
- Other commitments

Emotional Challenges

There are emotional elements that can be incapacitating. Each member may be faced with these at different times throughout the stages of care, no matter how well-equipped they feel.

- Grief
- Overwhelm
- Denial
- Resentment
- Stress

Personal Challenges

Also, you're an adult now with your own biases, beliefs, experiences, and even perhaps an agenda for what you would like to see happen.

- Biases
- Beliefs
- Experiences
- Agenda

Family Dynamics

Family dynamics are one of the biggest challenges of all and yet, one of the biggest opportunities. They offer us a roadmap for discovering some of the false beliefs from childhood that may have undermined our happiness in life. Many unresolved issues or childhood misunderstandings may be viewed differently as an adult, given the time to reflect.

Caregiving provides an opportunity to heal old wounds and strengthen a sense of belonging and unified purpose. In fact, creating a *culture of unity* is one of the defining principles of learning how to have a successful family conversation.

Perhaps you don't have a good relationship with your parent. Issues can be diverse and range from innocent expectations that caused a rift growing up, to more serious events such as childhood abuse. You may not get along with a sibling or have an old feud going on that is still smoldering. Every family is complicated in its own way.

- Relationship to parent
- Relationship to siblings
- Unresolved issues from the past

Sitting on the sidelines is no longer an option when it comes to working together as a family to make important decisions that affect everyone.

How Does a Family Stay Focused and Productive?

Structure is key for achieving consistent results and maintaining focus. You'll witness that each family member's capacity to participate fully will vary throughout the many years of care. This may encompass everything from grief and anxiety to overwhelm or being distracted by other personal commitments. Being able to follow a guide with steps that contain clear objectives is essential. In fact, a guide is like a neutral third party that keeps everyone on track and focused on the objectives, rather than on personalities.

Being diligent in following each step will help you to accomplish several important goals.

- **Objectivity** is essential for making good decisions.
- **Staying focused** on your loved one instead of each other keeps the conversation **productive.**
- **Measurable results** can be achieved by following a **repeatable method** and is important for understanding how to make necessary adjustments.
- **Improve outcomes** by consistently building on good information and incremental successes.

As you discuss needs, explore options, make decisions and create your plan, you will not only find new ways to interact as adults, but you may also heal old wounds without a word.

Look, Mom, no more therapy!

Know What You're There For

When you meet, have a clear agenda with all the information required to keep things moving forward. Areas to be discussed will involve:

- Medical decisions
- Legal decisions
- Financial decisions
- Residential options
- Support for all areas

Come With an Open Heart

Empty your cup before starting, stay focused on what you're there for, and accept that everyone has a piece of the puzzle. This is true no matter how much each might be struggling professionally, lack experience in a specific area or be inherently shy to comment. Each member will have something valuable to offer and a different perspective to consider. To circumvent or edit the full participation of any member is to undermine the process necessary to identify the best solutions.

It's also important not to allow hope or fear to drive your decisions. Decisions should be based on facts while keeping a firm grip on the reality of what is happening from day to day. *Reality-based thinking* is another important principle of good decision-making. Having methods in place to guide you during the conversation keeps things on track. Once issues are properly identified, responding with actionable insights is needed for maintaining your loved one's quality of life.

Try not to focus on fairness, something you probably fought for as siblings throughout your whole life. Focus instead on what you can contribute and how to solve the problem at hand. What matters now is not what you feel, it's what you *do*. You don't want to look back with regret, but rather with pride for the choices you made, and also for the kindness you showed in less than perfect circumstances. You may find that the kindness you show in tough times can heal your heart more completely than looking for others to heal it for you.

What Legacy Will You Leave Behind?

You also have an opportunity as a family to build your legacy. Your children are watching and learning by example what it means to be a family and what love really is. How you practice the **Guiding Principles** of love, compassion, empathy, acceptance, and service to family under challenging circumstances will guide them through the rest of their lives.

"So powerful is the light of unity that it can illuminate the whole earth."

Baha'u'llah

Your priorities when family needs you show what you stand for. You can be a beacon of light or just someone who focuses rather on their own needs when things get tough. Showing up for family is much more about who you are than how deserving your family may be of your support. What you do may or may not change your relationships, but it will definitely change you.

Pause and Reflect

- Staying objective is the family's biggest challenge.

- Everyone has something valuable to contribute.

- Everyone will have challenges at some point. Don't rely on fairness! Instead, focus on the issue and how to get things done.

- Every family is complicated. However, kindness is one of the most powerful qualities you can share during challenging times.

Remember the Guiding Principles and decide what legacy you want to leave behind.

Learn about how to make good decisions as a family. Take the Conversation Course NOW!
@caregivingoutloud.com

Chapter 4
Put Safety Practices in Place

"It isn't what we say or think that defines us, but what we do."
- **Jane Austen**

Safety, What Are You Waiting For?

Did you know that falls are the number one cause leading to premature death of the elderly? Safety is one of the easiest and cheapest things to do, yet it's one of the most common things people look back on with deep regret if not addressed. When a fall does happen, we all wonder why didn't we do something sooner.

Of course, everyone has good intentions. But good intentions are not the same as taking the necessary steps to avoid a crisis. It's easy to deny signs of decline. That's why **the checklist** is your best friend and your closest ally for establishing safe practices. It is an objective tool for staying on top of things. Rely on the checklist instead of your memory to keep your loved one safe. It's amazing how often people need to experience an actual crisis in order to realize the importance of being proactive.

I'm here to sound the alarm for you to put the necessary practices in place *before* (instead of after) something catastrophic happens. At some point, falls will happen, unless you intervene. They can happen at any stage; at home, at the hospital, and even at the best of care facilities. Continue to monitor for safety wherever they may be living.

My Story

Following a surgical procedure, my father was receiving physical therapy so that he could regain his strength and functionality. The process was painful and sometimes discouraging. Keeping him motivated was a day-to-day challenge. If he had given up at any point, he would never have been able to walk again.

As your loved one's advocate, it's important to stay engaged. Health challenges can reduce your loved one's ability to rebound, thereby reducing their quality of life. They need your ongoing support and encouragement.

At the nursing home following therapy one day, my father was left alone too long after lunch. He'd been waiting for at least two hours for someone to take him back to his room. We had all encouraged him to believe that he could start walking again. So, walking again was exactly what he did that day.

Frustrated by having to wait so long, Daddy stood up and began to walk for the first time, just like we all encouraged him to do. But we never expected him to try it on his own. He walked eleven steps before he fell, breaking his hip. No one imagined that he had the strength to get up from his wheelchair unassisted. And yet we all worked hard to convince him that he could do it!

What Could We Have Done Differently?

After the fall, my father never walked again. It would have been so easy to put a restraint on his chair to prevent such a tragic event. The pain he experienced was devastating. I still remember him screaming out as the nurse turned him over in his hospital bed one day after the event. I ran over to him and fell across his frail body, sobbing. He immediately tried to console me—imagine that. But then, that's love.

Daddy spiraled downward and died six months later. Had his fall not occurred, he could have lived several more years in significantly better health, continuing to engage with his surrounding community at the nursing home.

Loss of Independence

Nothing can circumvent a loved one's independence quicker than a fall. There are many reasons that falls happen, several of which may not be obvious until you really think about it.

If your loved one falls resulting in an injury or a subsequent concern serious enough to mention, you can safely assume that this is not the first time that it has happened. A senior has a lot to lose by admitting to a fall. Rarely will you learn about it directly from them. In fact, they may fall several times before you become aware of any problem. If you're not proactive, please realize that you are, in fact, waiting for something to happen before taking preventative measures. And then—as in my dad's case—it may be too late.

Let's talk about the key areas to watch for and how to mitigate the risks in each. There are three main areas to consider for safety practices:

- Home Environmental risk factors
- Physical risk factors
- Behavioral risk factors

The home environment is usually what we think of first. However, there are important physical and behavioral risk factors that need to be considered as well.

Assess the Home Risk Factors

Below are some areas to start with. However, everyone needs to do their own assessment and act according to their own personal situation.

- Declutter the house
- Remove obstacles/objects from stairs
- Check for adequate lighting
- Install safety bars in bathrooms
- Make sure to have nonslip surfaces
- Remove rugs
- Add handrails where needed

Assess the Physical Risk Factors

Consult a professional for a comprehensive **functional assessment** to determine your loved one's physical risk factors. Existing or developing physical issues can be identified and assessed for support, safety, and the assistance that may be needed to keep an emergency event from happening. Once you have addressed their current needs, you can monitor for changes in their condition and the need to reevaluate for additional support as your loved one declines.

Below are some examples of issues to be considered for a functional assessment:

- Gait
- Balance
- Mobility
- Vision
- Hearing
- Bathing

- Incontinence
- Urinary tract infections
- Medications
- Mental status
- Foot problems

Getting your loved one assessed and monitoring them closely are essential for avoiding unnecessary events. Everything needs to be addressed carefully. Seemingly small things can become the source of a bigger crisis, sending your loved one off to the emergency room.

Assess the Behavioral Risk Factors

Behavioral risk factors can be challenging to modify. Have you ever tried to go on a diet or improve your exercise habits? This is no different. Of course, the older we get, the harder it is.

Your loved one may need a cane or a walker to stay safe. And yet, they are not used to using one or keeping it nearby. This is especially true in the middle of the night when they have to go to the bathroom and may forget to use it. Or they may think that it's not that far to go, and misjudge their stability. Falls from nighttime bathroom trips are notoriously common.

No one wants to accept the loss of their independence or their encroaching decline. A lack of cooperation can be conscious or unconscious. There are many dynamic factors to consider and plan for. Going through the proper steps to carefully assess, consult, and address each concern is key to your success in keeping them safe. Don't forget to *reevaluate often* for changes in condition and environment! Noticing the small things can be tricky. You must be diligent!

The Bigger Picture

However, it's also important to evaluate their overall condition honestly and discuss what to expect over time with your loved one's primary doctor. If you spend thousands of dollars to implement safety projects at home without the real prospect of them staying at home, you may waste valuable resources that you will need for the later stages of care. This is an important reality check and a big decision. Hoping that your loved one is doing better than they are, or the fear of losing them one day, cannot be the basis upon which you make these important decisions. Identify the facts and let them guide the actions required to support your loved one's true needs.

It May Be Time for a Comprehensive Plan

You are embarking on a long journey. Getting the big picture as early as possible will help you make better day-to-day decisions as you go, with fewer mistakes. Remember that each decision will have an impact on the overall plan.

- How fast will your loved one decline?
- How long will your money last?
- How can you make sure they will have the best quality of life for as long as possible?

Most of us are doing this for the first time. I want you to learn from my mistakes, so you don't have to make the same ones that I made.

>Start with the **Safe at Home Program** @caregivingoutloud.com

Pause and Reflect

- Falls are the #1 cause of injury leading to premature death.

- Safety is cheap and easy to do.

- Don't wait for a crisis to do something!

- Your loved one may be hiding a developing issue for fear of the loss of their independence.

Think about what the environmental, physical and behavioral risk factors are for your loved one. And learn about the functional assessment in the Medical Module.

Chapter 5
Create a Comprehensive Plan

"Enjoy the little things, for one day you may look back and realize they were the big things."

- Robert Brault

How Do You Improve Outcomes?

A comprehensive plan is the most effective path toward mitigating the risks of caregiving while creating the best outcomes possible for everyone involved. This includes not only the loved one in need but also the family, and even the industry that is serving them. In fact, the process of planning itself helps you to understand in detail what will be required and how to get the support you need. Once in place, you will be ready for every stage of care.

Each decision made will have its own ripple effect, and each mistake can cost both you and your loved one dearly.

The "lovecare effect" is about creating an intelligent structure around care management that empowers you to achieve the best possible outcomes.

By using the system I created, the ripple effects I refer to can be anticipated, minimized, or even stopped before they create multiple downstream problems. The intelligent structure is founded on making good initial decisions, acting on them, measuring their effectiveness, and making the adjustments needed to stay on track by working optimally. Simple decisions can have a lasting impact. However, a lack of structure and the absence of good planning can create just the opposite—a domino effect of ongoing crises and poor outcomes. The list of things that can go wrong is surprisingly long and can seriously compromise what you hope to achieve. A key thing to remember is that all the areas of long-term care management are interconnected and dynamic, with each impacting the other. No decision or outcome happens in a vacuum. Each event influences many other things. That's why you can be blind-sided by this domino effect when even a seemingly small thing goes wrong.

It's critical to always keep your eye on the big picture when making even the smallest decisions. The purpose of the system is to guide you through an often, emotional process that is dynamic in nature, with simple steps and a check-and-balance method to measure everything you do.

Key areas you can mitigate by planning in advance:

- Family conflict
- Emotional turmoil
- Unnecessary costs
- Unnecessary crises
- Declining health
- Premature death
- Poor outcomes

Planning Now, Helps Avoid Conflict Later

Getting agreement up front once you've done your research helps the family to think through and discuss their options. The goal is to avoid potential arguments and blame when something gets missed or doesn't go as planned. However, you cannot mitigate all risks or stop the process of decline.

As I mentioned before, every family is complicated in its own way. That's why it's unrealistic to expect that everything will run perfectly all of the time. There will be unavoidable crises and unexpected events that will leave you at a loss, wondering what you might have done differently.

We all must accept our own humanness, as well as the reality of what is ultimately inevitable. We cannot save our loved one's life; we can only try to keep them as happy and as safe as possible while we still have them with us. To be successful, requires a comprehensive plan.

Taking the time to research, getting expert advice, and sharing all points of view allows a family to process what's going on and to learn over time how to manage what can be a heartbreaking process. Trying to cope under pressure and making snap decisions that may not work out, can build stress over time. This pressure can easily erupt into conflicts that can break a family apart if precautions are not taken.

Planning ahead not only reduces the probability of conflict, it teaches a family how to work together effectively, building bonds of love for an important legacy that each family member can look back on with pride.

Financial Mistakes Can End up Coming Out of YOUR Pocket

Most people have too much money to qualify for government assistance, but not enough to pay for long-term care. If you have a finite amount of money to spend on long-term care and don't want it to come out of your own pocket, plan ahead.

"Fifty-seven percent of women are more worried about running out of money in retirement than dying."
> - *The Allianz Women, Money, and Power Study: Empowered and Underserved, 2011*

You can easily spend money unwittingly without a comprehensive plan. This mistake can also rob your loved one of the quality of life they deserve and could have had, had you just planned for it.

Planning ahead also helps you to understand the big picture. When you plan ahead you can see the impact of each decision in the overall scheme of things and minimize potential mistakes. In addition, you are able to take the time necessary to do proper research, discuss the information, and weigh the pros and cons before committing to a course of action. Planning in advance allows for more objectivity and therefore, better decisions versus reacting to crises as they happen.

Mitigate the Risks of Spiraling Down

Caregiving can be stressful even when you plan ahead. If you don't, what happened to me may happen to you, too. I went from an 11,000 square foot home to a reluctant, yet thankful move into my boyfriend's apartment. If you're in denial that this is a real possibility, I can assure you it is.

However, life can fall apart on many levels before you ever realize it. If you are not paying close attention, you may experience a gradual spiraling down, an evolving snowball that often starts with grief. For me, it ended with not only the loss of my father, but the loss of everything I owned.

Emotional health can easily impact your physical health. Again, in my case, the more depressed I got, the more I stayed in bed. The more I stayed in bed, the more weight I gained. As I gained weight, I became insulin resistant. I went from working out two-and-a-half hours a day to never leaving the house unless I had to.

Women providing nine hours or more of caregiving per day:

– Are six times more likely to suffer depression[1]
– Have double the risk of coronary heart disease[1]
– Are more likely to also suffer from[2]**:**

- Emotional stress, anger, and anxiety
- Exhaustion
- Reduced immunities
- Increased substance abuse
- Poor physical health
- Higher mortality rates

[1]Long-Term Care Financing Reform: Lessons from U.S. and Abroad, Howard Gleckman, 2010
[2]Family Caregiver Alliance, 2012 and Senior Care Services, 2012 NFM-9103AO.1 (08/12)

Avoiding Crises

Part of planning ahead is staying ahead of your loved one's decline. From knowing what to expect throughout the stages of decline to anticipating the financial expenditures, you can avoid many unnecessary crises. Lack of medical planning may compromise your loved one's quality of life or even shorten it. Monitoring their needs closely allows you to be proactive instead of reacting to an avoidable event. Many steps can be taken to keep them safe by just planning and monitoring carefully. However, when a crisis does occur, you can be ready for it with planned options that can be implemented quickly.

Achieving Best Outcomes

Planning ahead is your primary tool for achieving the best outcomes for everyone concerned. The more you plan, the more everyone can enjoy a more normal life while taking care of a loved one in need. The less you plan—letting things just happen—the more chaotic your lives may be, and the less likely your loved one will thrive in their remaining years.

Planning ahead allows you to use this precious time to bond as a family. It can teach you what to look for, how things work, and who can help you when you need it. It allows your family to learn how to work together and to discover that their differences can be valued as unique strengths instead of weaknesses given time.

Family is at the core of who we are. You may find that the process of planning can be healing for you and your family on many levels. Unfortunately, the lack of planning can be equally destructive.

Love is in the details …

Pause and Reflect

- Rely on the intelligent structure you create to improve outcomes rather than emotion.

- Only an end-to-end plan can give you the comprehensive oversight for such a dynamic and long-term challenge.

- A lack of planning will produce poorer decisions, poorer outcomes and unnecessary crises wasting time and money.

- A comprehensive plan mitigates risks in every area including medical, financial, legal and emotional.

Details matter!

Take the Planning Courses NOW and Create your Comprehensive Plan!

@caregivingoutloud.com

Chapter 6
How Does Cognitive Dissonance Threaten Our Success?

"We see things not as they are, but as we are."

- Anais Nin

What Is Cognitive Dissonance?

Cognitive dissonance is the existence of conflicting beliefs or behaviors. This conflict creates a mental discomfort that must be resolved by altering one or the other. For caregivers, the knowledge that a loved one is in decline and the unwillingness to accept this fact as reality, creates a cognitive dissonance for them that can have a dramatic impact throughout all stages of care.

These conflicting realities between what is actually happening with what we want to happen, can only be resolved in one of two ways: by changing your belief or changing your behavior. But there is also one other way we use to cope: denying that anything is happening at all. Looking for a sense of comfort in the face of this cruel inevitability, we may tell ourselves that things are better than they actually are. This false belief is what sustains us. To change it is to give up and to accept that there is nothing that we can do, when in fact there is nothing further from the truth.

The journey between the challenges you face and what you do about them is in fact, what nurtures the journey of transformation.

The Short Trip from Cognitive Dissonance to Denial

We are all familiar with the five stages of grief when someone dies. In caregiving, your loved one has not died, but is instead aging over time. For this reason, denial is an ongoing battle that must be fought daily. It is a coping mechanism for something that is too painful to accept. To pretend that it's not happening gives us temporary relief from this discomfort, but at the same time, increases the threat to our loved one who may not get the care that they deserve.

Since we can never fully resolve the dissonance of losing someone we love, changing our beliefs is almost impossible. We can, however, act on a new belief, that every step we take can lead to improving their daily life.

How Does Denial Affect Our Loved One's Care?

Denial starts by ignoring or minimizing the first signs of decline.

If you are saying to yourself, *Oh, it was just a fender bender* or *Everyone forgets things,* you may be endangering your loved one's safety. However, not wanting to accept that one day you will lose them, is human. We all do it.

You would think that this initial process would demonstrate the importance of being proactive. However, denial continues to creep back into every stage of their decline, shielding us from the looming reality of what's to come. But it also impedes our ability to think clearly and to respond to our loved one's needs. Every change in condition is an affirmation of what we fear most. Managing grief is one of the main challenges that caregivers face, and is integral to making good decisions along the way.

How Does Dissonance and Denial Affect Decision-Making?

When dissonance becomes too painful, we fall back into a state of denial. We become emotional and sometimes even irrational. In this state, making decisions can no longer be objective or methodical.

So, fighting dissonance and denial is especially important during the many times when decisions have to be made. Will they be based on hope or facts? As your loved one declines, each decision will either support their increasing needs or perhaps shorten their life by ignoring them.

How Do You Combat Dissonance and Denial?

Dissonance and denial are combatted by facts. Going through a series of fact-based questions is the intervention necessary to keep you and your family on track. You will be making decisions often as you plan and manage the process together over time.

This fact-based sequence offers the **reality check** needed to combat the denial that can interfere with evaluating things objectively. If done emotionally it will not give you the results you hope for.

Managing the decision-making process within a broader context or plan can help to change behaviors over time.

Get the **How to Make Good Decisions Guide** in the **Conversation Course @caregivingoutloud.com**

Watch Out for the Downward Spiral

In my personal experience, worry and anxiety only produce more worry and anxiety. However, focusing on your worst fears can initiate an emotional downward spiral if you're not careful.

I've found that the best way to break this cycle is through an intervention. Think for a minute what the best possible intervention might be—one that you could turn to over and over again to get things back on track. One that you can count on for direction and consistent results. One that gives you confidence. The best intervention that you can turn to for keeping everyone on the right track no matter what swirling emotions or dire circumstances, is the comprehensive plan you are now creating.

If you plan in advance and follow the steps for making good decisions consistently, your comprehensive plan will become the best resource that you can turn to whenever you feel lost, overwhelmed or confused about what to do next. Even when you want to pretend it's not happening, your plan will always be there for you and your family to follow as a guide, putting distance between emotion and the actions necessary to support your loved one. What better tool could there be than the one you have already agreed on as a family, and spent hours researching and discussing?

Cultivate Your Spiral Upward

While the downside of operating emotionally is generally poorer outcomes, harnessing these misguided emotions can be used to gain important insights. Emotional energy can be utilized instead to transform what feels like hardship into new meaning and purpose.

We have all seen this happen to people when they experience a natural disaster. As we see victims on TV sharing their stories of fear and heartbreak, their story inevitably evolves into the gratitude they feel for being alive. Right before our eyes, we witness them changing their focus from the transient things in life to the more meaningful, such as family.

When faced with the possibility of death, we see over and over that the most human reaction is to begin asking the **"meaning of life"** questions like ... *Who am I? Why am I here? What is my purpose in life?*

During the course of caregiving, you may find yourself asking these same questions more than once over the long period you'll potentially spend isolated and perhaps even alone. Caregiving is not a disaster that happens suddenly and then ends, where the healing starts immediately, and you begin to move on. Your loved one hasn't died. Instead, they're in decline for an indeterminate amount of time. Your own life now hangs in the balance as well. What will you do with it? You may experience a sense of incremental loss over time—and turn inward for answers. This is how caregiving offers us such amazing opportunities not only for change, but for true transformation.

"The pilgrim resolves that the one who returns will not be the same person as the one who set out."
                         - **Andrew Schelling,** *(Meeting the Buddha)*

Neither hope nor denial are strategies that will help you to achieve the best outcomes for your loved one. However, a well-thought-out plan, using a system of checks and balances, can keep you consistently on track.

Learn why the checklist is so important in **Chapter 7.**

Pause and Reflect

- Dissonance and denial are a constant battle when caring for a loved one.

- Denial offers temporary relief but creates inaction and impedes the process.

- Denial interferes with the objectivity needed to make good decisions.

- Act on the belief that everything you do can improve the quality of life of your loved one in spite of the inevitable.

Think about the ways you may be unconsciously in denial. Is it depriving your loved one of the care and assistance they may be needing?

Chapter 7
The Checklist

"Start by doing what's necessary, then do what's possible, and suddenly you are doing the impossible."
- Francis of Assisi

Why Is the Checklist So Important to the Caregiver?

Ah yes, the checklist! As I mentioned before, the checklist is the caregiver's most trusted friend.

No matter what the circumstance, it can transform chaos into order. It can offer you a hierarchy of importance in a dire situation, a set of simple steps for a complicated task. It shows you the big picture at a glance when you are overwhelmed and suggests a place to start if you feel paralyzed.

NASA has a checklist 10 feet tall. If the smartest people on the planet need a checklist, maybe caregivers do too. When astronauts leave the earth embarking on a new frontier not knowing what to expect; they plan in advance for all the possible risks and desired outcomes. Could they reach their objectives without a plan? How is caregiving any different?

A checklist is like an outline of either necessary or possible things to do or consider. Even astronauts understand that they can't keep everything in their heads. What if they forget something important? What if they each remember something differently? What if what they forget could have saved their life? What if they don't accomplish their mission?

Astronauts going into space are not the only ones who use checklists. Pilots here on earth use a checklist every time they take off and every time they land, even though they may fly every day. They especially need it in an emergency when things happen unexpectedly. Firefighters use a checklist to make sure they've packed the truck correctly with everything they need before they go out on a call.

We may think that if a checklist contains simple or obvious items, that we don't need it. You never think you need a checklist until you forget something really important. The more obvious it is, the more you end up kicking yourself, and of course explaining to the others that although you had a checklist, you decided not to use it.

But the checklist is also part of something bigger. It's actually the first step in creating your entire action plan where you begin to gather information, develop a scope of work and determine what support you may need. While emotion stops the ability to act, the checklist focuses your attention so that emotion and overwhelm dissipate, and you can function more effectively.

The checklist also gives you an immediate context for what's at hand. You may feel lost and don't know where to start, just like Dana. Dana was a project manager working for the military. In fact, she taught project management. Even though she specialized in the step-by-step management of projects, under the stress and emotion of her father's sudden hospitalization, she could not apply what she knew and used every day in her work. She came to me confused and frustrated trying to express how overwhelmed and powerless she felt.

Here's one of the many texts Dana sent to me:

> **Jun 17, 4:30 PM**
>
> **Hey Lee, my dad's in the hospital. Had the dreaded family care planning meeting, "moment of truth" reality check, his-care-is-in-your-hands kind of thing yesterday, and I thought of you: "What would Lee do?" I've got to get a handle on all of this. How in the world did you do this alone for 15 years?? I'm disoriented if I could put a word to what I felt yesterday. Any advice?**

What got Dana back on track? We started with a simple checklist to get organized for what she needed to do in that moment. In one second, she went from overwhelmed and lost to clear and in control again. She was ready.

What small thing could spiral out of control that may put your loved one's life at risk? A magazine left on the floor, not drinking enough water, or maybe waiting too long for that eye exam? Any one of these could cause a fall or a sudden change in condition that could worsen their quality of life or even lead to a premature death.

How can the checklist improve **your life?**

More Ways a Checklist can Help You

- A checklist can make things efficient, helping to avoid costly do-overs.

- A checklist can help to coordinate with others, giving you an organized method for dividing tasks, moving through a project, and keeping everyone on track.

- It allows you to do things the same way each time so that you can measure your effectiveness.

- It helps you to combat the denial you feel that your loved one is declining by taking the important actions necessary.

- It improves outcomes.

In fact, I would say that caregivers have a very special case for needing the checklist more than anyone. Why? Because professionals who use checklists approach whatever they do unemotionally, with a clear understanding of the essential role objectivity plays in achieving their mission. For caregivers, it's always personal.

How Do You Stay Objective?

However, since caregiving is emotional by nature, we have to constantly mitigate the risk of allowing it to stagnate our efforts or interfere with our judgment.

Just like a doctor never operates on their own family, it's almost impossible for a caregiver to be unemotional. Objectivity is a constant challenge for many reasons.

Reasons Why It's Hard to Stay Objective Checklist

- ☐ **Family Dynamics** - The process of making decisions can trigger old resentments or conflicts, making the process less productive and perhaps even flawed.

- ☐ **Denial** - Denial is insidious and can take many forms, keeping you from acting in time to prevent a crisis.

- ☐ **Fear** - The fear of losing someone you love and what that means can cause you to lose focus on maintaining their best quality of life.

- ☐ **Overwhelm** - Overwhelm can paralyze you from taking any action at all.

- ☐ **Sadness** - Sadness can cause you to spiral downward, impacting your own health.

- ☐ **Personal Bias** - Personal bias can influence your decision-making rather than relying on facts.

- ☐ **Limited Experience** - You don't know what you don't know. Without proper guidance, you can easily miss important things or fail to connect the dots.

Until now there has been no comprehensive training for caregivers and in fact, little recognition of their significant challenges. They are often seen as incidental to the process, if not invisible.

So, for us caregivers, the checklist is the first tool you grab out of the toolbox. It can be extrapolated and expanded into infinite detail for anything that needs to be implemented. All good action plans start here.

- ☐ **Lack of Preparation** - The last but most important item on our checklist of reasons why it's hard to be objective, is lack of preparation. When you are prepared by researching, taking time to process, and getting input from everyone, you can overcome almost everything else.

How Do You Measure Your Effectiveness?

If you do not have a process that you follow each time, you cannot measure the effectiveness of what you are doing. If you cannot measure the effectiveness of what you are doing, you could be wasting valuable time and money, not to mention the opportunity to make things better for your loved one.

Each area that you will have to manage, from tracking your loved one's condition to tracking their finances will require what?
Ah yes... a checklist!

In fact, all good outcomes start with the often misunderstood and underestimated checklist. However, you will soon find out that the lowly checklist may turn out to be the #1 tool in your toolbox.

Pause and Reflect

- The checklist is your most objective tool in the toolbox. It is the #1 way to combat dissonance and denial.

- Don't take its simplicity for granted.

- The checklist helps you to focus, unifies everyone, offers efficiency and a way to measure your effectiveness.

- The checklist is the foundation for everything else you will do.

Get in the habit of doing what the professionals do. Depend on your checklist, not your memory.

The Checklist

Find complete checklist instructions for

Decluttering, Homecare Set Up, Moves and Selling the Home @caregivingoutloud.com

Chapter 8
Questions to Ask Yourself Before Becoming the Primary Caregiver

"Circumstances don't make you; they reveal who you are." -
James Allen

Know What You're Getting Yourself Into

A caregiver is a person who takes primary responsibility for the logistics and affairs of caring for a loved one through every stage of the aging or disease process, the duration of which could last from between one to fifteen years. While this challenge brings with it many gifts, it also comes at a cost. If unprepared, a caregiver can lose their job, their marriage, their home, and even their health. That's exactly what happened to me.

However, with the right planning and tools, caregiving can be one of the most important and rewarding things you ever do.

By 2030, 20 percent of the U.S. population will be 65 or over. During the same period, the number of 85-year-olds will increase by more than 50 percent, and the number of 100-year-olds will nearly triple. However, the number of nursing homes is falling. (*Data for this section were compiled primarily from Internet releases of the U.S. Census Bureau and the National Center for Health Statistics/Health Data Interactive*).

The lack of preparedness shows us that even though 10,000 people are turning 65 every day and living on average 18 years longer, we somehow think that our own parents are exempt from this inevitable statistic. The reality of this trend is life-changing, affecting how you may spend the next 10-15 years of your life.

The New York State Office of Aging states that 50% of family caregivers will be caring for a loved one for at least five years, 30% for five to nine years, 14% for ten to nineteen years and five percent for 20+ years.

In light of these staggering statistics, assessing your strengths and weaknesses is essential for determining whether you're comfortable taking on the responsibility of caring for your loved one. If you do not assess your strengths and weaknesses honestly, you could be heading for disaster. This affects not only you, but your entire family. Unfortunately, it's not a decision that is easily reversible. You must be truthful with yourself about your capacity to do what's needed and be ready to do it for a very long time.

Questions to Ask Yourself

- Do you have a sufficient support system?
- Does your job allow the flexibility to respond to repetitious crises?
- Do you feel comfortable assisting your loved one with daily care? (Bathing, dressing, administering medications, incontinence needs.)
- Are you physically capable of lifting on a daily basis?
- Are you emotionally capable of handling stress and grief over an extended period of time?
- Do you have any addictions?
- Can you manage your loved one's behavior based on your relationship?
- Do you have a strong marriage with good communication? Don't underestimate the toll caregiving can take on a marriage.

- Do you have the finances, time and skills that will allow you to handle this endeavor?
- How will an infirmed loved one affect your family and household?
- Do you have enough/appropriate space in your home?
- Can you administer suppositories, clean up vomit or change an adult brief?

These questions may seem basic or even obvious. Some may even be embarrassing to think about or discuss. However, facing the reality and scope of caregiving and what the commitment will mean to you and your family, is essential to consider before you say yes.

The Caregiver's Challenges

The challenges of disease are daunting for a patient. But what challenges do caregivers face over the years of caring for a loved one?

I became a caregiver when I was 15. My mother had cancer. She was bedridden for five-and-a-half years before she died. This was my first experience as a caregiver, although it would not be my last.

You can read my poem about cancer and what it taught me @caregivingoutloud.com

Many say that quality of life has not yet caught up with the extended quantity of life that has been achieved. I wonder if we have really absorbed what this means to families who are responsible for their parent's care now that the elderly population is living longer, but not necessarily better.

Based on my experience, I think that the call to action for this new normal has revealed an even deeper level of love, responsibility, and commitment to family. I've seen individuals who, although taken by surprise and without adequate finances, embraced the challenge right away. They seemed to be compelled by something more than just the relationship itself. I discovered that it was more about who they were and the principles they believed in rather than the relationship—good or bad—that they had with their loved one. As a result, their lives shifted dramatically in some very positive ways because they stepped up and did what was necessary.

Dana's Story

> Hey cuz im trying to reach out to you because your dad is very ill and has been admitted to the hospital. So call me and tell your brother...

This was Dana's **surprise phone call!**

Dana was dropping by the hospital out of duty for a quick visit. But that quick visit turned into a commitment that she knew would last for the rest of his life and a substantial part of her own. Although Dana's father had never been there for her growing up, she didn't hesitate to take on the responsibility of caring for him, knowing that it would be hers and hers alone. How do you explain this?

> I'm grateful for these extended moments. I told Daddy that I had been trying to figure out for years how to get back to being his number one girl and now I am.

At first, as you can see by her text, that she was still haunted by the unresolved need for her father's approval, perhaps the unconscious but motivating force behind her decision. Torn between a long-held anger and yet the need for his love, she drops everything and begins an unexpected journey that will change her life.

Dana had not seen her father for many years, avoiding him because of the hurtful history they had together. But in the midst of all these swirling emotions, Dana had to decide where she stood, not only with her father, but more so with her own values. She could stand in the shadows of the past or she could follow her principles when they counted the most. She chose to take care of him.

But caring for her father would not be her only challenge. The emotions that she began to feel after making this decision, exposed the open wounds that had never healed, tormenting her as if it were yesterday.

You may be thinking that Dana made a mistake by allowing herself to become so vulnerable, once again. But this is the power of choosing to become the primary caregiver rather than watching from the sidelines. This was Dana's opportunity to heal and to live her life in the present instead of stuck in the past. Making this decision, although her father died before he could leave the hospital, was an utter leap of faith. On some level Dana knew the emotional issues she would have to face, and yet she did it anyway.

> ‹ Messages (1) **Dana**
>
> Goodmorning Lee, I started vomiting yesterday but not a lot came out. The nausea hit me all of a sudden and wiped me clean out. I got the sweats, really strong cramps and extremely agitated. I was a hot mess. I thought it was all mental at first and felt anger, sadness, frustration, distrust and fear. Although I

This text reveals the depth of how affected she was by the history they shared.

It took a while for her to absorb what was happening. I witnessed Dana, finally shedding that little desperate girl seeking Daddy's approval. She shared how it had affected her since childhood living every day with fear and anxiety, robbing her of a normal adulthood.

In the last days of his life, she stopped needing to work for his love. By having the courage to face her fears, Dana finally got to experience the greatest gift a parent can give to their child, unconditional love. This was the moment that changed her life. She finally felt what it was like to be loved simply for who she was. Dana was finally free.

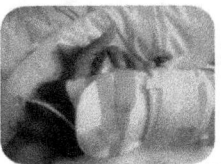

If I could use one picture to sum up what this whole experience has been for me so far, it would be this...

In the end, it was her courage that won her freedom. That's why caregiving is such a hero's journey.

As I said before, every family is complicated in its own way. And everyone has to decide what's really important in life, when it's their turn.

Pause and Reflect

- Be honest with yourself about your strengths and weaknesses before deciding on whether to become the Primary Caregiver.

- Remember that caregiving takes planning.

- Although it's a huge responsibility, it's one that's worth it.

Find out what the primary caregiver needs to know before deciding, in the Planning Course.

Chapter 9
A Change in Perspective

"One's destination is never a place, but rather a new way of looking at things."

– Henry Miller

Changing Your Perspective Changes Your Experience

The easiest way to mitigate the creep of negative thinking is to view each situation as an opportunity to see things in a different way. This is not only a psychological practice that caregivers need to adopt, but also a spiritual one that offers more positive options for how to deal with day-to-day challenges.

How Can a Change in Perspective Help You?

We know how important it is to build personal resilience. This includes creating good habits that ensure good mental hygiene. What is good mental hygiene?

Let's use a familiar metaphor. Imagine keeping your closet perfectly organized, free of clothes that don't fit anymore and tossing out old worn shoes. As soon as you notice something out of place, you straighten it; you donate an outfit you haven't worn in years. You inspect and discard what is no longer wanted regularly. You know exactly where to find whatever you need. This metaphor is also an example of how to support good mental hygiene; a clean way of living where you can function more freely, reducing life's daily chaos and leaving more mental space for thinking, planning and just being.

If the closet I just described was your brain, the regular "spring cleaning" would help you to achieve more perspective during times of emotional clutter. Perspective, or outlook, is a very proactive tool—one that you can utilize daily.

I'm not referring to putting on a happy face or trying to maintain a positive attitude. Perspective is a courageous, conscious, life decision to find value in every circumstance, no matter how negative it may appear to be at the time. In fact, it's in the worst times that we often gain the most insight and momentum to take great leaps forward.

"You cannot control what happens to you, but you can control your attitude toward what happens to you, and in that you will be mastering change rather than allowing it to master you."

- Sri Ram

What is Wabi Sabi?

The Japanese have a term called Wabi Sabi, based on the acceptance that life is transient and imperfect. This concept holds a high place in Japanese culture. Richard Powell states, "Wabi Sabi nurtures all that is authentic by acknowledging three simple realities: nothing lasts, nothing is finished, and nothing is perfect." The Japanese find beauty in imperfect things such as placing a higher value on an older teacup that shows the patina of the years rather than a new one out of the box.

For caregivers who face difficult realities every day, this important mental pivot can have a life-changing impact.

Making the Perspective Pivot

"When we are no longer able to change a situation, we are challenged to change ourselves."

- *Viktor Frankl*

How Can a Change in Perspective Help Your Loved One?

Imagine that after a few years, you see your father's dementia begin to worsen. He now forgets which room is which. It's sad to watch, and you fear he is declining at a faster rate. Even though you may be sad, get into the habit of creating a new normal out of an imperfect circumstance.

Look for solutions that focus on living rather than on declining. If he forgets which room is which, so what! Post signs: bathroom, bedroom, sitting room, kitchen. Make life normal again until it's time to create another new normal. Find the joy in sharing the everyday things. You will never run out of "new normals" with the right perspective.

You can change perspective on the spot about almost anything. One time in the nursing home, my father and I were sitting in the TV room watching a show. I was trying to get him to eat his dinner. He turned to me with an impish grin and said, "I hate you."

It was so out of character for my father, with whom I had an incredibly close and loving relationship, it was actually funny. I could have reacted with wounded anger, gotten up and left or any other number of other negative things that could have initiated an unfortunate snowball rolling in the wrong direction.

Instead, I looked at him in total surprise and laughed out loud, saying, "Okay, take another bite and hate me some more." Then we laughed together at what could have turned out quite differently. Instead, it became another reason for growing closer instead of growing apart.

Challenge yourself to look at difficult situations differently. You can flip so many potentially hurtful events simply by responding differently with a change in perspective.

How Do You Consistently React in a Positive Way?

If your focus is on how things affect YOU, caregiving may be difficult. But if your focus is on solving problems, having compassion for others, and achieving good outcomes for your loved one, this change in perspective could begin to change your life.

Listen for Information

Listening for information allows you to stay focused on what's at hand versus how you feel about it. Listening with the goal of learning how you can add value—even if it's just to listen—allows you to be an objective observer. Reacting emotionally can change a potential course correction to a lost opportunity.

Every situation affects you in one way or another, but the best solution for most problems is usually what's best for everyone involved. Ask yourself how you can contribute to solutions instead of focusing on what's wrong. If you use this approach, listening for information and focusing on practical solutions, day-to-day problems will be more easily resolved.

How Can a Change in Perspective Help Your Relationships?

Imagine that your sister arrives from out of town. You're the primary caregiver. Because she is remote, she has contributed little to your father's care. She criticizes everything you do, even though she hasn't participated in his care at all. You could easily justify reacting with anger. But instead, listen for information and try to understand why your sister feels the need to criticize the only person actually taking responsibility for his care.

You may realize that behind her criticism lurks a sense of guilt for not doing more. You may discover her sense of feeling powerless, living so far away and wishing that she could contribute somehow. However, she thinks that she can only participate by finding and commenting on things that she perceives need to be improved upon. While you don't have compassion for her criticism, you can have compassion for her feelings of guilt over not being there to help.

How Can the Perspective Pivot Change Outcomes?

You might try responding to her criticism by asking her what she thinks would work better. Tell her that she might have a more objective perspective not being there every day and not dealing with the situation on a daily basis the way you are doing. Come up with something that she could help you do remotely and ask for her participation. This might make her feel more included and more useful in the process.

These small but powerful shifts in response to a negative attack can transform a potentially volatile situation into a bonding interchange without an emotional confrontation, if done from the heart. The power that a loving response can have is immeasurable to a family undergoing long-term stress. And, it is never forgotten.

Listening for information is a habit that can be cultivated. It can flip a negative situation into one with an extremely positive outcome. It can unify a family going through hardship. It can even heal old wounds without a single word.

Pause and Reflect

- Remember Wabi Sabi! Appreciate the imperfection in life. Nothing lasts, nothing is finished and nothing is perfect.

- Our own perspective is the one thing we can control.

- A change in perspective can help you to pivot to what works.

- A different response based on a change in perspective can be healing to everyone.

Remember to always listen for information instead of reacting emotionally.

Chapter 10
Start Monitoring Your Loved One Early

"Life is about choices. Some we regret. Some we're proud of. We are what we choose to be."

- Graham Brown

Know What to Expect and Be Ready for It

What causes the most stress during caregiving?

In all my conversations with caregivers, they always tell me that it's worrying about the unknowns. From what to expect medically to wondering if their money will last, these are the issues that keep them up at night if they haven't planned in advance.

Planning in advance will answer most of these questions ahead of time, positioning you for a state of readiness with a range of options for when sudden events happen. Being prepared ahead of time with answers to these critical questions is key to maintaining a more objective, effective, and less stressful caregiving experience.

Although you cannot plan for everything, knowing what to expect and being able to respond successfully will build confidence over time for both you and your family. You will be able to handle surprises and become increasingly proud of the job you're doing every day. Those who aren't prepared for the range of possibilities that may come next and what to do about them, set up a never-ending game of Whack-a-Mole, creating poorer outcomes for everyone. If reacting to things as they happen *is* your approach, you may not be aware of the complex challenges caregiving requires. It's never too late to plan forward.

What is Monitoring?

The most effective solution I've found for mitigating the unknowns is by simply creating a good **monitoring plan**. Monitoring your loved one is the number one tool that can help you to anticipate the myriad of avoidable complications that you may face throughout long-term care. It's the key to making the incremental adjustments necessary to achieve the highest quality of life during every transition of your loved one's decline.

Monitoring also alerts you to the *"transition triggers"* presented as either tipping points or sudden changes in condition that warrant increased care and a possible move. Because these events can happen suddenly, if you're not prepared, they can set off a whirlwind of critical decisions that must be made quickly. This can lead to overwhelm and conflict within a family if not managed well. Imagine how different it would be if all these decisions were agreed upon in advance, and everyone stood ready to play their part instead of fighting about what to do and who's to blame.

To boil it down simply, every time there's a change in condition, there's either a need for an incremental adjustment or a potential move for increased care. From the initial surprise phone call to the end stage of life, caregivers must recognize the varied signs indicating the need for reevaluating their loved one's needs to ensure safety, health, and quality of life for each stage of care.

It's vital to know when your loved one needs further assistance as they decline. Monitoring is the centerpiece of what you will rely on most for tracking these changes in condition, whether incremental or abrupt. Monitoring is also the key to the **actionable insights** that make the difference between poor outcomes that you may regret and improved outcomes that everyone can celebrate.

What are other Reasons Why Monitoring is So Important?

Monitoring your loved one's rate of decline gives you a critical window of time in which to plan in advance for their developing needs. This helps you to avoid having to make snap decisions during a crisis.

Monitoring also allows you to gauge the success of your current care plan and daily routine, alerting you to incremental adjustments and ongoing needs as your loved one's condition evolves. Measurable metrics allow you to reevaluate how well your current plan is working and if anything needs further scrutiny.

Monitoring alerts you when it's time to call the doctor and signals the need to initiate the downstream process of implementing a major transition for increased care. **Think of monitoring as the DNA for achieving better outcomes for your loved one.**

However, another important person to monitor is you, the caregiver. What's happening to your own health and well-being during these challenging years? How are you coping? Are you spiraling up with successful methods and insightful *aha* moments, or spiraling down in overwhelm? Grief, stress, family dynamics, and isolation can all take their toll. You cannot take care of your loved one if you're not taking care of yourself.

What are the Ways Monitoring Can Help You?

Monitoring is all about increasing your ability to be **proactive.** However, you must maintain vigilance by identifying, measuring, analyzing, making improvements or adjustments, and uncovering additional needs that require attention.

Being Proactive is Important to:

- Plan effectively and efficiently
- Maintain your loved one's best quality of life
- Maintain you and your family's best quality of life
- Discern threats as early as possible
- Avoid crises
- Prevent conflict
- Build trust and confidence with loved one/family
- Avoid unnecessary expenditures and mistakes impacting long-term funding for care

The Cost of Doing Nothing

- Unnecessary crises
- Conflict
- Poor decisions/outcomes
- Avoidable trauma leading to the premature death of loved one
- Loss of time, money, relationships, job and peace of mind
- Overwhelm, stress, depression, declining health of the caregiver

When Do You Start Monitoring?

Minor observations of decline, age, health, or mental status should alert you to begin the process of monitoring your loved one's risk for events or complications that may suddenly arise or worsen. Be proactive! Each medical evaluation will inform you of a projected time frame to prepare for future but inevitable changes. You should start by asking the "Big Questions."

Find out more about the **"Big Questions"** in the **Monitoring Module** @ **caregivingoutloud.com**

Move Early

Evaluating the need for assistance is key to maintaining quality of life. Early assistance should be the norm, rather than the exception when planning ahead. We need to wake up and be proactive instead of waiting for a crisis. In hindsight, it's always obvious that waiting for a crisis is the *absolute worst* possible caregiving strategy there is and yet, we all do it.

Below is a guide for transitional moves based on typical care and assistance needs.

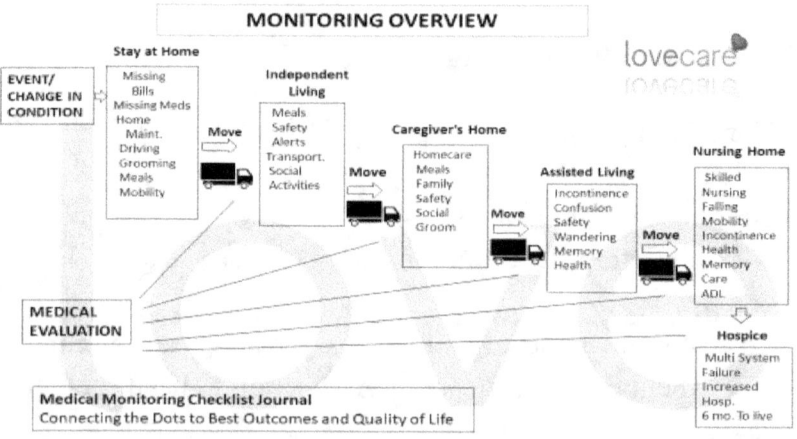

Monitoring Through Stages of Decline

It's important to remember that insights from the primary caregiver are extremely valuable in piecing together your loved one's evolving health puzzle. You are the only one who will have the big picture of your loved one's condition. You will always have the best vantage point for connecting the dots, noticing the subtle changes and linking issues or events that may not be considered properly without your input. Never be afraid to share your observations and insights with the doctor.

Start Monitoring Your Loved One Early

Types of Medical Monitoring (Refer to the full Monitoring Checklists)

- Mental (affairs management, memory, wandering)
- Emotional (anxiety, depression, engagement, signs of abuse)
- Physical (mobility, grooming, health)

The Challenges of Early Monitoring

Monitoring should begin early while at home, well before any significant change in condition develops. This allows you to proactively watch for signs of decline which may trigger the need for additional assistance to prevent an unnecessary event. But although this is one of the most important times to monitor, it is also one of the most sensitive and poses a potential threat to a loved one's independence. However, you don't want to look back with regret and wonder why you waited.

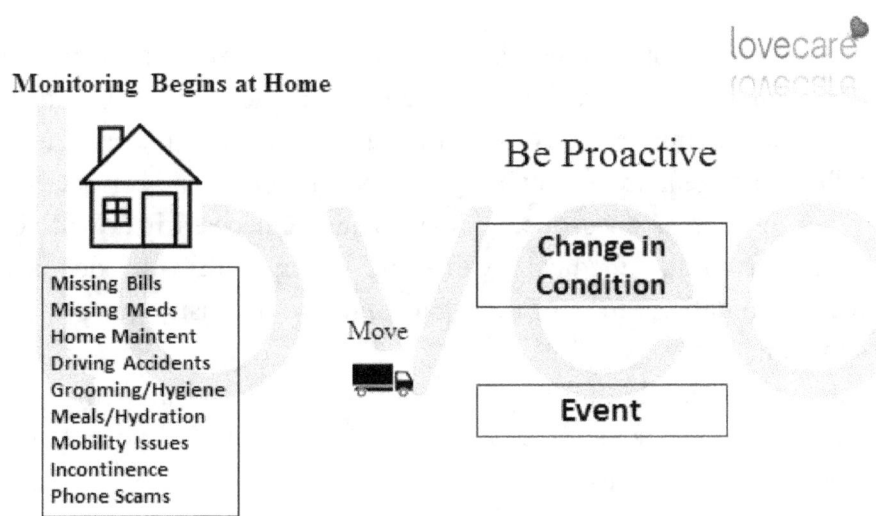

Although maintaining independence is important, the best way to preserve it is by catching signs of decline early before an event occurs. You don't want them to be robbed of the additional years of independence they could have enjoyed if not for an incident that could have been avoided.

Many falls go unreported for fear of losing independence prematurely. A loved one may fall several times before getting hurt and requiring assistance. Approach this as a partnership, agreeing on incremental steps to keep them safe while giving them the assistance they need to maintain their independence for as long as possible.

However, changes in condition can happen suddenly. Also, signs of decline can go undetected since they happen slowly over a period of time, making it difficult to notice changes if you're not watching closely. Minor things such as not getting to the bathroom in time can turn into a catastrophic event like a fall, from which they might never recover.

On the other hand, minor issues like urinary tract infections are often mistakenly perceived as signs of dementia because they manifest as similar states of confusion. What may appear to be a radical change in mental stability may be temporary and correctable. When a change does occur, don't panic unnecessarily. Wait for results from the medical evaluation, along with your doctor's recommendations to confirm what might be an easily correctable situation.

Just understand that all issues need to be addressed proactively if you are to keep your loved one safe and healthy and you off the emotional roller coaster.

You may think by now that I am repeating myself. You are right! But life is precious, and we cannot get it back once it is gone.

Medical Advocacy

It's always important for you to be present at every medical appointment in order to have a clear firsthand understanding of your loved one's current condition and needs. Knowing the details will allow you to make incremental adjustments and establish new markers from which to measure future changes. Your doctor has many patients, and your parent may not remember or volunteer news that might endanger their independence if they are currently living on their own.

Start early and stay on top of things!

Driving is another important area of concern, one of the "Big Questions" you'll need to be asking that will significantly impact your loved one's ability to function on their own. These are difficult issues and tricky to navigate. I discuss how to approach these difficult conversations, pitfalls, and resistance strategies in more detail in the **Conversation Course.**

For more info on the Conversation Course, go to caregivingoutloud.com

The best solution is to be proactive and get agreement to stop driving early. Invest in a transportation service. Waiting for a fender bender is unnecessarily dangerous. Your loved one will probably not give up driving until an accident occurs and they're forced to stop. Giving up the keys to the car is a turning point and one of the most significant losses of independence in a line of many to follow. Make transportation options easy and attractive to keep them safe.

As a caregiver, you want to avoid the **surprise phone call.** Catch crises before they happen by monitoring and being proactive.

Remember: Have regular checkups and monitor like their life depends on it!

Pause and Reflect

- Monitoring is your #1 best mitigating tool to catch concerns before they turn into crises.

- It is the DNA for achieving better outcomes.

- Monitoring keeps your life more predictable.

- Remember, diligence is key.

Make sure your loved one has regular checkups. When was their last check up?

Learn how to set up your monitoring plan in the Monitoring Module.

Chapter 11
Understanding the Big Picture

"Doctors diagnose, nurses heal, and caregivers make sense of it all."

- **Brett H. Lewis**

The Big Picture Puts the Smaller Decisions into Context

It's important to take the 10 steps back we all need to see the bigger picture. We are often too busy or distracted to connect the dots of our loved one's condition without the help of some good tools.

The jigsaw puzzle is a great metaphor for monitoring—by putting seemingly unrelated signs of decline together it can show us a bigger picture that can reveal a new trend evolving. The ability to observe subtle changes allows you to intervene early preventing them from worsening. The ability to step back will give you the actionable insights needed to help you achieve better outcomes.

The ability to step back offers important opportunities to:

- Notice and understand cause and effect
- Span the medical gaps between doctors
- Avert unnecessary crises
- Maintain best quality of life
- Improve outcomes
- Keep **your** life more predictable

By gaining actionable insights you can, unlike a puzzle, actually change the big picture. In fact, by seeing trends and patterns developing, you can make the needed adjustments before a crisis occurs.

- Stop a trend from becoming a bigger issue
- Preserve quality of life
- Prevent the snowball effect from happening
- Prevent an emergency

Cause and Effect

You may be able to connect the dots between two seemingly unrelated items to stop a developing trend. By stepping back, you may observe that the days your loved one takes a certain medication they get dizzy, or that the days they feel depressed are days when you're not there. The ability to view relational data can reveal a lot of important conditions that may be happening under the radar impacting their decline. If you spot them, you can do something about them.

How Do You Span the Medical Gaps?

Your ability to connect the dots and share your insights with your loved one's doctors is invaluable. You are their advocate and their voice. In my experience, doctors are typically more focused on their main specialty. You must be able to broaden their view and give them the bigger picture of what's happening in other areas, so that they have all the pertinent facts to make more informed decisions.

How Do You Avert Crises?

An observation can turn into a complaint, a complaint into a concern, a concern into an issue, and an issue into a completely avoidable event had you been able to step back and identify a developing trend. It's much easier to avert a crisis when you can catch a problem early.

How Do You Maintain Quality of Life?

The best gift you can give your loved one is the most optimal quality of life for as long as possible. This requires small adjustments and proactive steps to prevent issues from worsening. Incremental adjustments are key to your loved one's comfort and happiness in all areas whether mental, emotional, spiritual, or physical. To see the big picture, you have to look at the whole person. Understanding this can have a dramatic impact on their overall well-being.

How Do You Improve Outcomes?

Improving outcomes takes a dynamic view of the interrelated elements of care. Having the capacity to step back gives you this view. Seeing how disparate elements evolve over time and intervening before they reach a tipping point can make a huge difference in improving outcomes. Incremental adjustments can also have a big impact on the comfort and safety of your loved one. Improving outcomes is the only real measurement that matters.

How Do You Keep Your Life Predictable?

Your life is busy. Two of the most valuable things a system can offer you and your family is predictability and peace of mind. Having the tools to evaluate what's happening and what needs to be done gives you the confidence that you can do your best job and still enjoy your own life. When you can see not only what needs to be done but also understand the impact it will have overall, your loved one is safer, and your life becomes more predictable. Better decisions can prevent costly do-overs saving both time and money.

Predictability allows you and your family to enjoy a more normal life during the very challenging years of caring for your loved one.

Pause and Reflect

- Remember, as the primary caregiver, you are the one who has to make sense of it all.

- How will you keep your eye on the big picture?

- How will you prevent crises from happening?

- How will you improve outcomes consistently?

Put your plan in place so you can manage the details while keeping your eye on the big picture.

Go to caregivingoutloud.com to find out more about the Grab & Go APP

- Fingertip management for long term care
- Spot trends by viewing relational data
- Team coordination
- Everything all in one place

Chapter 12
Be "Option Ready"

"It is in your moments of decision that your destiny is shaped."
- Tony Robbins

Why is Planning in Advance the Answer?

Part of your comprehensive plan is to have all your transition options ready to go for all future stages of care as your loved one's needs increase. This includes all of the projects, moves, and purchases required to execute each transition. Knowing exactly where your loved one will go based on their evolving condition, who will help you, and what it all will cost to implement is what I call being **"option ready."**

You may not know exactly when or what specific condition will unfold, but you can be armed and ready to respond with the appropriate solution for an evolving situation at a moment's notice. The time it takes to research, cost out, and plan for each stage of care is involved and cannot be postponed until the last minute. Hurrying under pressure is how mistakes are made and valuable assets can be unnecessarily wasted without proper time to research and discuss ahead of time. If you make quick decisions that don't work out as hoped, you may find yourself in a do-over. Do-overs also take a dramatic toll on your loved one, depending on the circumstances

My Story: The Do-Over

I got a call one day from the Assisted Living Facility where my father was living. He had fallen a few times, none of which had been serious. But because of the additional care required, they could no longer allow him to remain in their facility. For me, this was one of the surprise phone calls that I never expected. They gave me three days to find a new solution. I quickly moved my father into what I thought was a stellar nursing home close by. Many well-known people had their parents there, and according to the reviews it seemed like a great choice.

However, I noticed that there were only a few windows and only one small awkward area where the residents could go outside. Although the care itself was excellent, within a very few days, my father started to go downhill psychologically. I actually thought I was going to lose him. I scrambled to visit the one other nursing home on my list, which I had skipped due to the narrow time frame in which I had to make a decision.

Although it was an hour-and-a-half away, it was beautiful. There was a lake and a gazebo where Daddy and I would eventually spend many long afternoons together having lunch and feeding the swans. The staff was great, the food was wonderful, and the space was expansive. They had a robust activity agenda, and church every Sunday. The minute I saw it, I knew what a big mistake I had made. I had been in such a rush because I wasn't **option ready.**

I sat with the manager of the new facility and tried my best not to cry, although unsuccessfully. I knew that the waiting list was over six months. I was so afraid I would say the wrong thing, and my father couldn't wait. I begged her to take him. Luckily, there was a shared room that had just become available, and thankfully she offered it to us. I was in shock, but I had made up my mind that I wasn't leaving without a room for my father.

His new roommate was a man who happened to be an engineer, just like Daddy. His wife had become an expert in creating the **"new normals"** that kept a declining life more manageable. One day I walked in to see she and her husband (who had Parkinson's), eating ice cream cones as if it were a Sunday afternoon at home on the front porch in Georgia. He was reading the paper. The only problem was that it was upside down. Did she care? No!! This was their own new normal that made life work. What a perfect match for my father. Whew! Daddy moved in the next day.

This was a miracle, and I was lucky. With fewer and fewer nursing homes being built, fewer available nurses, and 10,000 people turning 65 every day, you may not be as lucky as I was, unless you plan in advance.

I truly believe that my father would not have survived another week. Although he never complained, I can only surmise that when he saw what felt like a room full of warehoused seniors, he just gave up. When that happens, it's possible to lose your loved one very quickly.

I could feel it, and I had to act fast. He thrived at the new location, but if I had planned in advance, this costly do-over would have never happened. The last thing you want is to look back with regret, knowing that you could have done something different had you only planned in advance.

Stay Engaged

I could tell by his condition that Daddy's feeling of well-being coincided with the number of visits I made each week. If he didn't see me every other day, he would become despondent. In truth, I probably needed to see him even more than he needed to see me. I discovered a new gym on my rather long drive to visit him, so that I would not neglect my own "well-being". I began working out more regularly than ever before. Remember, there is always a positive way forward if you look for it!

I knew how critical my regular visits had become, and I made sure that I never missed one, no matter what. As time went by, sometimes I would stand behind one of the columns before he knew I was there, looking to see if he was happy. As I stood there, I watched him staring into space, lay his head down on the table, and then look back up from time to time.

It was so sad to see my father like this. How could anyone really be happy away from home, away from the life they used to have? But the minute I came around the column and he lifted his head up and saw me, his face came alive and there he was again—my beautiful father, full of love… and everything was okay again. At least until it was time for me to go.

Pause and Reflect

- Is it safe for your loved one to be living at home?

- What safety projects will you need to consider?

- What equipment or professional services might help them?

- Where will they live during each stage of care?

Make sure you don't get caught with costly do overs. Plan ahead and be Option Ready!

Chapter 13
Organize Your Team

"Family is not an important thing. It's everything."

- Michael J. Fox

If You Want Support, You Better Be Organized

As a caregiver myself, to say that I had no team is an understatement. I was lost the whole time, going from one crisis to another. For me, the isolation of caregiving on my own became the beginning of a downward spiral.

But you don't have to suffer through the same mistakes I made. You can assemble your team way ahead of time. A team can help you build confidence and establish an effective routine. In fact, establishing roles and responsibilities is part of the lovecare planning process. It gives you great peace of mind knowing that you have people who are standing by you to help with each stage of care.

- **Half of adult caregivers say it's moderately or very difficult to balance work and caregiving.**
- **Three-quarters of respondents found it to be stressful, and more than half found it to be overwhelming.**
- **Depression affects 20 to 40% of all caregivers.** (Caregiver Burnout, Updated 2022, Aging in Place.org)

Disparate Support Can Create Desperation

The beauty of a comprehensive approach is that disparate information is transformed into an end-to-end plan and the disparate care continuum silos are transformed into a team sharing the same dynamic system. What was separate, is now one process. The efficient coordination and ease of having everything in one place changes the experience for all stakeholders, from the patient, to the family, to the industry that serves them, and especially for the caregiver. Numerous gaps are closed and achieving better outcomes becomes a shared goal that is much easier to attain.

This is what lovecare is all about: integrating family caregiving into everyday life.

Replace Isolation with Organization

To maintain a team, whether it's family and friends, doctors and professionals, or service providers and vendors, you have to be organized.

- ✓ Know what you need
- ✓ Know when you need it
- ✓ Know who can provide it
- ✓ Have all current information at your fingertips

Knowing exactly where everything is and being ready takes the stress out of worrying about what you're going to do, not *if*, but *when* something happens. Having a team is also a great emotional support. Since we're all doing this for the first time, we can't be experts at everything. It's a relief to know that someone has your back in every area.

Be Prepared When You Meet Your Team

It's important to have a clear understanding of your loved one's needs, and exactly what services you will require to address them. The less you know, the more each professional will have to charge. If you don't understand the process, it will be difficult to reign in unnecessary services to keep your costs manageable. You can save a significant amount of money if you educate yourself and are prepared with your loved one's information. Following blindly from crisis to crisis leaves you vulnerable to unnecessary expenditures and companies that may not have the expertise they claim to. Take the time to research carefully. Costs add up fast.

The best professionals will also have more respect for you if you are organized with targeted questions. They will see you more as a valuable partner instead of a damsel in distress.

Crisis or just being unprepared will cost you!

Be Honest About Strengths and Weaknesses

It's critical to be honest about people's strengths and weaknesses. If you are not, you'll set yourself up for failure. Whether it's a family member or a professional, if they can't provide what you need, you'll experience a breakdown in your support system when you need it the most. This is paramount to understand, especially when it comes to family. With family, there's more at stake than just getting the job done.

Pick the Right Person for the Job

A sibling may not be a numbers person, but instead may be the most compassionate and loving member of the family. Another sibling may not want to change an adult diaper but can manage a move with no problem. Some of you may have a better relationship than others with your loved one. Compensate without judgment for each other's weaknesses, and you will have a great team.

Judgment makes us focus on where each is weak, but love is what makes us see that our differences are in fact, our greatest strengths.

Pause and Reflect

- Get organized by planning everything in advance.

- Build your team now so that they are ready to respond.

- Don't get caught trying to caregive alone.

Go to the Support Module in the Planning Course to build your team! Our coaches are there to help you.

Chapter 14
Building Resilience for the Caregiving Marathon

"The most minute transformation is like a pebble dropped into a still lake. The ripples spread out endlessly".

— **Emmanuel**

How Do Small Changes Create Big Momentum?

If you cannot maintain your own well-being, you will not be able to manage the well-being of your loved one. The need for resilience is never more critical than when caregiving over the long term. Caregiving is not a sprint; it's a marathon.

We have talked about monitoring as the key to your loved one's medical resilience. For the caregiver, resilience is needed in every area. Resilience is not only important physically, emotionally, mentally, and spiritually, it's also important to develop financial and legal resilience as well. But building resilience takes planning.

Who Do You Want to Be at the End of Caregiving?

I am a good example of why building resilience is so important. After 15 years of caregiving my father, I had lost my business, my house, my marriage, and even my car. I was depressed, overweight, insulin resistant and alone, except for my dogs. But eventually, I started writing and then spent the next 10 years creating lovecare, so that you would not have to make the same mistakes I made.

All of us have different levels of experience in different areas. Almost none of us have deep experience in all the areas that caregiving requires. After all, most of us are doing this for the first time.

The saying, "You don't know what you don't know," is never truer than in caregiving. Why? Because it appears to be so straightforward. We think we can just manage it as we go. We don't take into account the debilitating emotions or the family dynamics that interfere with our ability to think clearly. The cognitive dissonance of dealing with loss pervades every stage of care, impeding your ability to stay objective or to even remember the most obvious things.

I invite you to take this opportunity to mitigate all these risks of long-term caregiving on the front end. I can tell you from experience, you will avoid a lot of heartache.

How Do You Create Personal Resilience?

Personal resilience starts with a well-thought-out daily routine. You don't have to do a lot, but you do have to do it consistently. From a few minutes of meditation to a quick prayer before rising, a few stretches, or even some qi gong exercises, small efforts can create meaningful momentum very quickly.

The "lovecare effect" is all about how to make the small changes that have such a big impact.

The impact of a daily routine is immeasurable when dealing with grief, family dynamics, and the daily stresses of caregiving. It's like making your bed every day. If you start with one consistent thing that you are committed to, even something as simple as making your bed, like it says in Admiral McRaven's book, you can change the world.

There is no doubt that you will have challenges at one point or another. But the resilience you build now will serve you well for rebounding quicker, pivoting more easily, and preventing you from drowning in the many events and responsibilities that will become your new normal.

It's not about How You Feel

It's important to understand that consistency is not dependent upon how you feel; it's about doing something *no matter* how you feel. On any given day you may be up, down, enthused, discouraged, energetic, withdrawn, happy, or depressed. If you act or don't act based on your feelings, you'll never create the momentum you need to achieve consistent results. When everything around you feels like chaos, your ability to be consistent in your practices can stabilize your life and steady your physical and emotional well-being, because tomorrow you'll have to get up and do it all over again. Make sure your tank stays full!

Learn How to Create Your Own Resilience Routine @ caregivingoutloud.com

Processing emotions as you go is critical for developing personal resilience. Grief, isolation, and family dynamics can take their toll and build up over time. These are significant areas that will drain your energy if you're not careful. It's very easy to put emotions on the back burner. We all do it, but processing the grief you feel on a regular basis and surrendering your daily fears and resentments, are essential for maintaining good emotional hygiene.

The goal here is to simply **let it go.** There is no doubt that there are deeper issues triggered by interactions that are potentially much more complicated. But analysis is never ending and you will find yourself just going down the rabbit hole. Focus instead on the daily practices that keep you in balance.

Let Go of Old Emotions

If old feelings of anger or resentment surface, it's important to understand that when it comes to family, no amount of talking will ever fully resolve the issue. Everyone remembers things differently and sibling rivalry is just part of nature. These deep wounds are never solved intellectually. They must be healed from inside the heart. When you change your focus from your own hurt feelings to having compassion for the hurt of someone else, it can transform an argument on the spot. Opening your heart, when it's the hardest, offers a powerful healing force that can often melt away the most impossible barriers to restoring a loving relationship.

Surrender

The act of surrendering has magic in it. As you surrender a seemingly insurmountable wound, your heart starts to open a little more each time. Regardless of whether it heals those around you, you will feel a weight being lifted and a surprising feeling of love pouring into the space left behind. More than once I have seen the deepest hurts melt away in an instant during which I felt like I was witnessing a miracle.

Empty Your Cup

Empty your cup every morning and surrender each day. This one simple practice will help you to let go of whatever happened yesterday and other things in the past that may be bothering you.

Whatever stress or disappointment… just let it go. By doing this you make room for a new day and living in the **present moment.** The present moment is the only time when you can actually change anything. Personal resilience starts by emptying your cup each and every day.

How Do You Create Family Resilience?

You achieve it with methods that keep your decision-making objective are critical. Objectivity helps you make good decisions and improve outcomes. Repeatable methods help you to measure what you're doing so that you can make the needed adjustments necessary. Using a dependable process will help you to build a foundation of trust and confidence between you and your support team. Processes allow you to learn as you go and to look back with pride on what you created together, even during challenging times. These strategies create the infrastructure that allow your family to build a legacy for generations to come. Without good methods, you may find yourself reacting blindly to events as they happen, hoping for a successful outcome and inadvertently setting yourselves up for failure and regret.

When it comes to family, failure is not an option!

What Are the Guiding Principles?

The **Guiding Principles** found in the **Conversation Course** and the **Self-Care Course** are excellent sources to help families refocus on what's really important, especially when things get personal. They give families the resilience they need for the long term. You will find that if you focus on fairness in caregiving, things will get even more stressful. Instead, fill the gaps by focusing on what needs to get done versus who is supposed to be doing it.

Each member will be challenged differently at different times. Each will have their own strengths and weaknesses. At any given moment, each one may experience their own denial, overwhelm, or confusion—all of which could compromise their ability to contribute equally. Some may experience family conflicts, work conflicts, or just not want to face the responsibility on any particular day.

The Guiding Principles prioritize love and service over fairness, acceptance over judgment, empathy and compassion over resentment. The Guiding Principles are not only key to reducing conflict, they are integral to expanding the heart during one of the hardest times you may experience in life. It's during challenging moments such as these that the process of transformation is accelerated.

"Looking back over a lifetime, you see that love was the answer to everything."

- Ray Bradbury

Learn more @ caregivingoutloud.com

How Do You Create Financial Resilience?

Financial resilience is key to everyone involved. Being a competent steward of your loved one's finances preserves their ability to pay for the best care they can afford and deserve. But it's also key to making sure that their care does not impact your financial well-being, and that of your immediate family. Mistakes and do-overs can be costly. Knowing what things cost throughout all stages of care and being ready with an overall plan is your best way to stay financially resilient and to successfully mitigate the financial risks.

How Do You Create Legal Resilience?

Legal resilience, like in other areas, is a matter of putting things in place ahead of time. Getting participation from your loved one is essential. Their wishes are paramount. However, at any point in time that you do not have proper legal authority to act on their behalf, everything stops. Legal authority is not easily resolved when you need it in an emergency. It can bring an abrupt halt to a critical need for action that can impact literally everything you need to do.

When conflict arises, things can deteriorate quickly. Having your loved one's legal affairs in order can help you avoid many disagreements that are hard to resolve. These disagreements can bring lasting disunity to an otherwise close family. Legal resilience is easy to achieve but can be very complicated to navigate if not carefully planned for ahead of time.

If you do not know what your loved one's wishes are from a medical point of view or their after-death requests, your family can be left with very disturbing struggles that may never be resolved to everyone's satisfaction. Lifelong trust can be challenged, and otherwise close relationships can sometimes be destroyed. Again, planning is the key.

How Does Resilience Help You Pivot?

If you are resilient, you can easily pivot to what might work better. Being resilient means that you've planned ahead and thought through other options if things don't go as expected. This makes everyone more open to discussing and sharing alternate points of view, building unity and trust along the way. Everyone can be engaged in a more natural flow versus reacting emotionally to an unanticipated surprise. It allows everyone to step back and gain insight about alternate ways to mitigate future issues. Resilience allows you to pivot, and the ability to pivot allows for progress to become more fluid.

For a loved one, it's the quality of care that determines their outcomes. For caregivers, it's the strength of their resilience.

Pause and Reflect

- Have you asked yourself what you can do to create the resilience you will need?

- What kind of a daily routine could you create?

- Do you have any old resentments you need to let go of?

- Make a habit to focus on solutions instead of what's wrong or personalities.

Create your Resilience Plan in the Resilience Training and Self-Care Course. Ask about the retreat.

Chapter 15
Plan the Funeral While Still Healthy

"Teach me your mood, Oh patient stars, Who climb each night, the ancient sky, leaving no shade, no scars, no trace of age, no fear to die."

- Ralph Waldo Emerson

The Last Chance to Make a Good Impression

Every one of us will need a funeral at some point. The question is, when will we plan it? Our collective response to this question is typically to put it off until the last possible moment—a moment that could not be more fraught with emotion.

Though most of us do it, this approach serves no one well.

The funeral can be an extraordinary moment of celebration for one of the most important people in our lives. Denying the fact that they, like each of us, will die one day robs us of the rich and wonderful experience the funeral can become. In fact, your loved one might want to participate in the planning of their own farewell.

The planning of a funeral isn't just a smart thing to do in advance; the earlier you do it the more meaningful you can make it. You might even say that although the funeral itself may not exactly be fun, the planning of it can be. It's not wrong to laugh about the dress you *don't* want to be buried in or ask for your favorite song to be played. This is an intimate and precious moment if shared with those you love, and a chance to remember the little things that are so important while your loved one is still alive.

The planning of a funeral can even be planned as a party of sorts for close friends who may also want to plan their own funerals too. (Of course, the final financial decisions should probably be left to the following day when the cocktails have been cleared away.) But just like making financial decisions after happy hour, waiting until your loved one passes is not the best time to plan a funeral.

Choose the Best Time for *You* to Plan

If you want to approach planning in a more sober environment, so to speak, there are two very natural and less emotional times you might consider. One could be during the legal conversation while discussing last wishes and critical conditions. Making funeral plans at this point can seem more like a natural last step in the sequence of dealing with the business at hand, initiated at the attorney's office and completed shortly thereafter as a family.

The second opportunity is during the financial conversation. The funeral is a one-time cost that needs to be considered in the overall budget. This expense is not a trivial one and needs to be researched and evaluated objectively. Although a very emotional task, it's an important purchase that shouldn't be made at one of your most vulnerable moments, at the point of need.

Even though the funeral may be an emotional subject, it should not be an emotional decision.

How Can Planning a Funeral Help You?

Getting funeral plans out of the way early can give everyone significant peace of mind. Waiting can feel like something is hanging over your head; you know you should do it, but you keep putting it off. You may also find that this is often a prepaid item that may help you loved one qualify for financial assistance if needed.

Regardless, you want to be focused on family when the time comes, not planning a funeral when your loved one has just passed away.

Initiate Your Memorial Plans Now

As you finalize your funeral plans, it usually brings up a lot of memories. Use this time to start collecting family treasures to remember your loved one by. When the funeral comes, you'll have a lot to share with friends and family to celebrate your loved one in a way that you can all be proud of.

I wish I had taken more pictures and captured more moments to remember my father by. You cannot easily recreate your time together after they're gone unless you collect those important moments along the way. It's so comforting for the whole family to have those "snapshots in time" to look back on, cherish, and pass on to generations to come.

Why Not Have a Funeral Party?

So, if funeral planning doesn't have to be a totally negative experience, what should it be instead? You can use this time as you plan your loved one's funeral to also plan your own. Create a fun, supportive environment to research and plan.

A little wine never hurts. In fact, bringing childhood photos, deciding on what you want to wear, what you want to be said about you and the music you would like, can be a fun walk down memory lane shared with close friends and family. Whether you decide on the Rolling Stones or Pachelbel, you might have a lot more fun than you think if you plan early.

Your loved one's input may even surprise you, given the opportunity. Planning the funeral could break the silence on other things that might never have been discussed in your family—things that could completely change your understanding and perspective about something in the past when heard from another's point of view.

Pause and Reflect

- Ask yourself if you are resistant to planning the funeral in advance?

- How could you make it memorable?

- What is the best environment for you to use that would be most comfortable?

Find out how to plan and how to get an apples-to-apples comparison in the Funeral Guide.

Chapter 16
Take Time to Heal

"Other things may change, but we start and end with family."
- Anthony Brandt

Looking Back

We've talked about the risks of long-term care and how to mitigate them. But there are no risks without some rewards.

Looking back, the grief and suffering I experienced over time turned out to be the process of an awakening to a completely new life. Hardship is a powerful experience that can, while at first may devastate you, can in the end make you stronger. I went from losing everything and being almost homeless after caring for my father to writing, developing this system, and now living in Greece.

As I mentioned before, many disaster survivors often gain a new perspective after experiencing severe loss and perhaps even a close encounter with death. Given this phenomenon, you could think of caregiving as a slow-moving disaster that unfolds day by day while experiencing the loss of a parent. But the miracle of the caregiving disaster is that it gives you more time to reflect, to integrate the experience and what it means. Pain brings with it important insights that can change your life. What seems like a devastating nightmare can instead become a second chance to find new meaning and new purpose.

As the tip of the spear, the caregiver cannot easily hide or turn away from the impact that loss brings. Those who are tested with this challenge cannot help but change. The question is how?

Going Back Home

"Going back home" is an opportunity to take a second look at things from an adult perspective, especially if you have had challenging relationships in your family growing up. Often, it's impossible to even remember what made us angry, yet we hold onto it our whole life. Sometimes things start with a simple misunderstanding from a child's point of view, which may not have even been an accurate account of what really happened.

You might have other things that are even more serious and harder to forgive and forget. But the process of coordinating with family during a challenging time can offer miraculous opportunities to transform the pain that you may have lived with your whole life.

As it turns out, caregiving forces us to face a perhaps buried past and to draw a line under it. This means that you're finished with being a victim of whatever happened. Letting go of it, what it has meant, and how it has defined you, is freeing. Instead of focusing on the seemingly impossible problem, a shift in focus to the bigger situation at hand amazingly begins the healing process. How? It's what I call the "bigger love". Making the "bigger love" a priority is what changes you. Your choice to take responsibility rather than to focus on the past shifts the whole paradigm from being a victim to serving the family.

We all feel an unspoken responsibility that comes naturally with being part of a family, no matter what has happened in the past. Whatever pain you may have grown up with and how it may have limited you in your life, often melts away as you rise above your personal feelings to help during a family challenge.

It is your response that changes everything going forward.

The Journey

This painful gift is a journey rich with opportunities for great leaps in awareness and self-understanding. When it's over, it has likely touched the core of who you are and who you will become. Caregiving is like nothing else I know, in that it combines courage and fear, love and pain, responsibility and surrender. It's an opportunity to see the reality of things, to reflect on our choices in times of challenge, and to see the truth of what we actually value.

However, what we experience only happens at the level we allow it. In fact, its significance is inextricably tied to whatever we can surrender to in the moment. We ourselves choose whether to suffer or to thrive. It is a courageous act to remain open and to trust life at our most vulnerable of times.

Letting go of your most prized illusions is hard. However, piercing the bubble of false beliefs that keep you from living life fully can restore you to the wholeness you deserve. Only truth can lead to a path of genuine freedom and happiness.

"A man travels the world over in search of what he needs and returns home to find it."

- George A. Moore

So, the answer to, *Who am I now?* is not based on just the loss of your loved one, but perhaps the loss of who you thought you were. It is the contrast of coping versus living. This period between the old self and the new can be scary or invigorating. Standing in that void can be one of the most creative times of your life, if you let it. This is what I refer to as *your* life after death. What you make of it is now up to you.

For me, caregiving was like an intervention saving me from myself. My own delusions were robbing me of being my whole self, and even more, who I could become.

"What the caterpillar thought was the end turned out to be the beginning of a new existence."

- Deepak Chopra

Choices

Caregiving reminds us how simple things really are. Every day you are faced with binary choices—responsibility or avoidance, acceptance or denial, love or fear, action or inaction. The choices you make tell the story. This rare clarity highlights the striking disparity of what should be easy decisions and why they can bring such strength or shame.

Where you stand on each will never be more important. Strength or shame add up every day, sending you spiraling up or spiraling down, revealing what you prioritize in life. There is no wiggle room in caregiving, no gray area to hide in. If you genuinely live your values, you do whatever it takes without weighing it in advance on how it will end up for you when it's all over.

Caregiving teaches us to trust life. It teaches us strength, tenacity, endurance, and responsibility in the face of the unknown. It changes you from the inside out and proves that no one else can show you your way on your own journey. If you don't find your own way, you will always be lost, asking others for directions.

The journey that began when you took on this important responsibility has now opened the door to a new reality, to new meaning. Loss simply clarifies what's important in life. This truth shines a light on your path going forward.

"Life can only be understood backwards, but it must be lived forwards."

- **Soren Kierkegaard**

Be careful not to squander this precious moment on sadness alone. The lessons will fade if you don't use what you've learned. Share them with other caregivers who may also be struggling. You are not the same person as before. Your new life will not be the same life as it used to be.

Reinventing Yourself

The need to reinvent yourself after caregiving is common. It's typically driven in mid-life by the search for more meaning rather than the need for more money. As we get older and have hopefully experienced our financial success, the passion to make a difference before we ourselves die, becomes paramount.

The death of a parent can drive home the reality that life doesn't last forever. Losing someone so close to you—a person responsible for your very existence, no matter what the history—can bring to the surface a question that you may have asked yourself at various pivotal points in your life. When you lose your job, get injured, get a divorce or when your kids leave home, *Who am I now?*

You may even start to reevaluate *What am I doing with my life?* If you believe that we are all here for a reason, finding that reason becomes more and more important as you age and discover that achieving material success is not the same thing as finding true meaning.

While challenges can make us stronger, clearer, and more present in the moment, caregiving is especially unique. The choice to embrace the "bigger love" brings with it a tidal wave so powerful that it can change what we have not been able to change for ourselves over a lifetime. Although the shift can be subtle, it is, in fact, a whole new approach to life, nurturing you spiritually and transforming you little by little until suddenly, you realize that the old wounds have somehow been healed and a new sense of freedom is now left in its place.

I asked the question at the beginning of the book, *Who do you want to be at the end of caregiving and what will it mean to you?*

How Will It Transform Your Life?

For me, I went from owning a manufacturing company to creating an end-to-end system for other caregivers like you, so that you would not have to make the same mistakes I made.

Will caregiving make your life seem harder or will it become the awakening that you need to find your life's true purpose?

You cannot deny what you discover during this experience; you can only choose to ignore it.

What Will You Do with What You Learn?

"Where the needs of the world and your talents cross, there lies your vocation."

- **Aristotle**

The Lovecare Effect

The death of someone we love can inspire us to discover what most of us seek at some point, *Why we all here ...*

That's exactly what happened for me. In the end, loss is what makes us realize how precious life is.

Caregivers, more than anyone, understand why the caged bird sings...

Pause and Reflect

- The need to reinvent yourself is common after caregiving.

- Don't waste this important experience on sadness alone.

- Loss can instigate meaning of life questions that can inspire new purpose.

- What will caregiving mean in your life?

What will you do with what you learn?

Start planning **NOW!**

An event could happen anytime and **YOU** could become a
CAREGIVER OVERNIGHT!

Planning is one thing you won't regret.

Start with the **Emergency Course**
@caregivingoutloud.com

If you are already a caregiver,
Plan Forward

BE READY!

www.ingramcontent.com/pod-product-compliance
Lightning Source LLC
Chambersburg PA
CBHW052148070526
44585CB00017B/2023